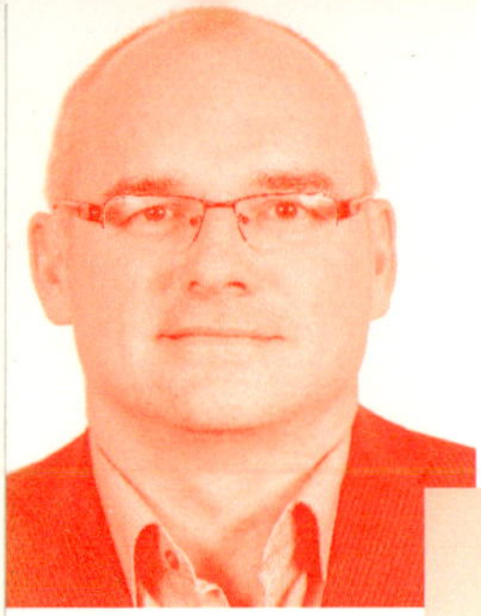
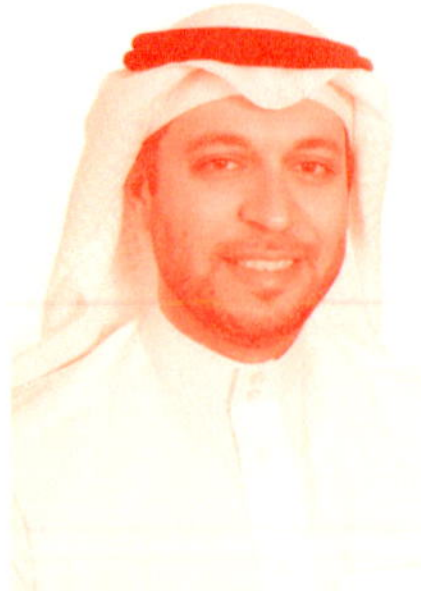
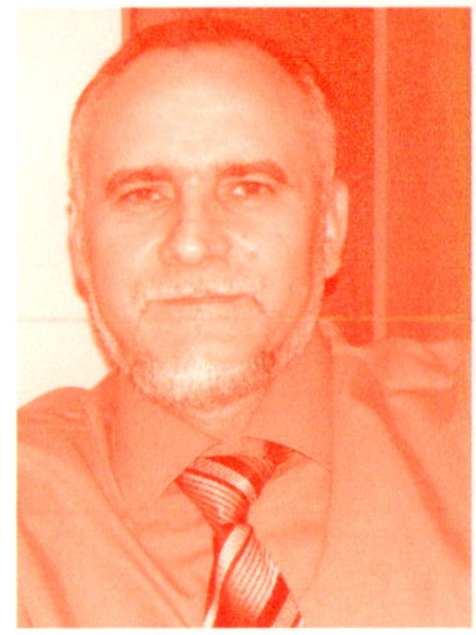
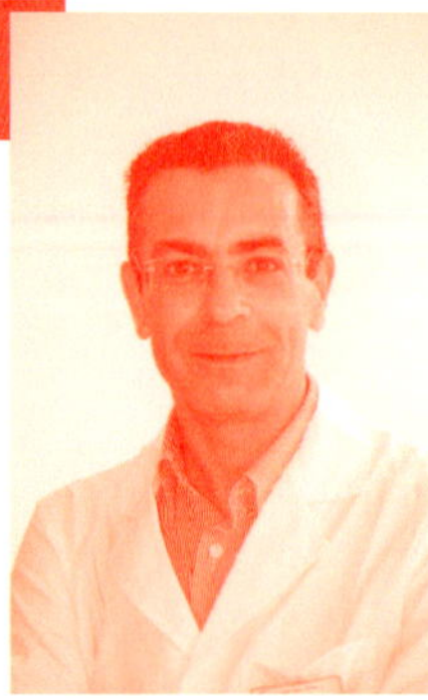
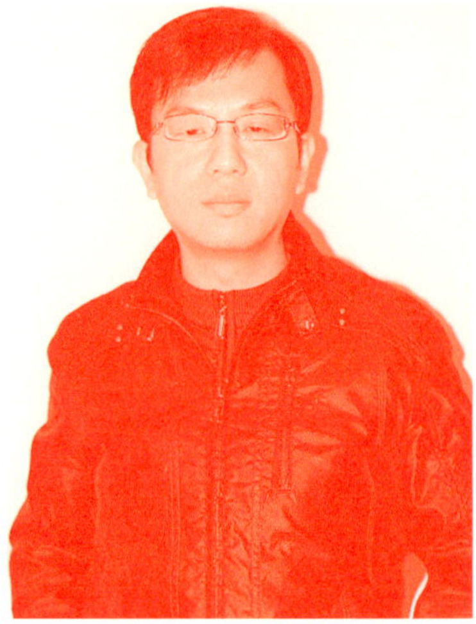
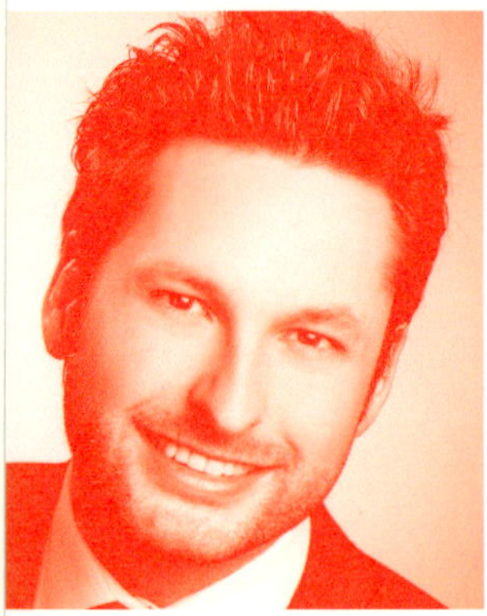
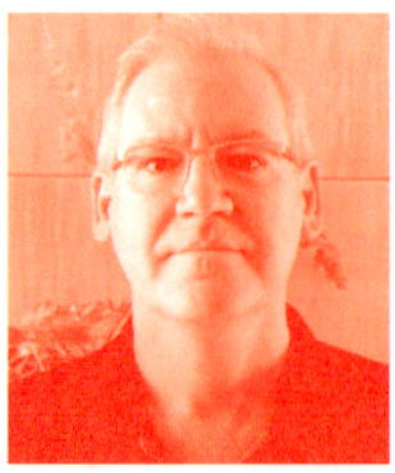

IntechOpen

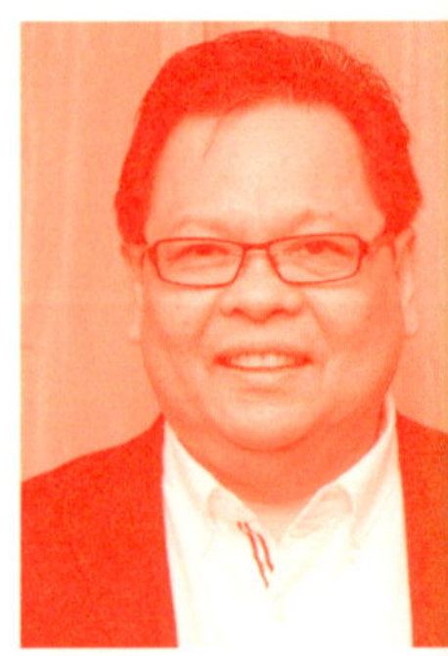
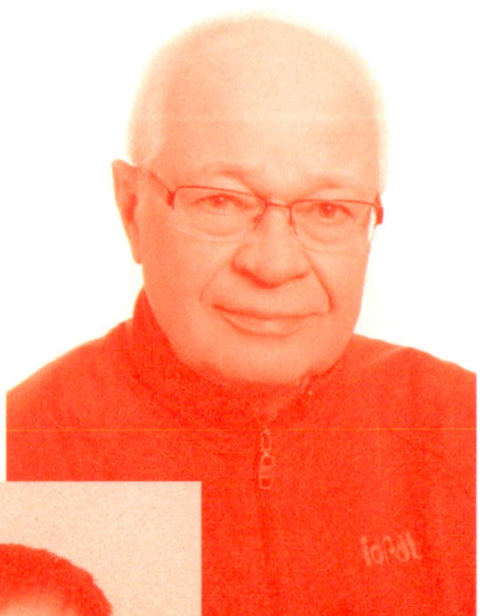
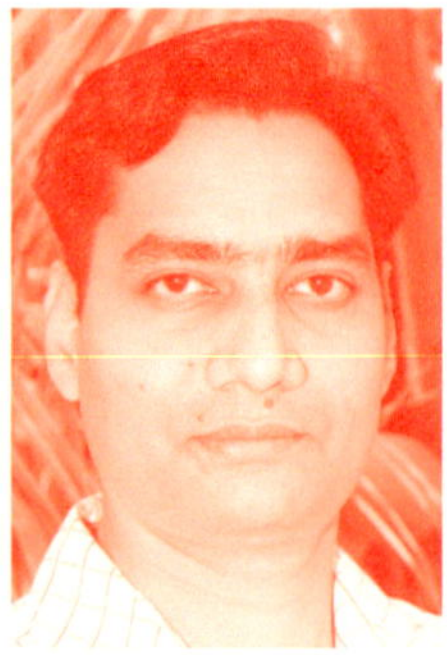
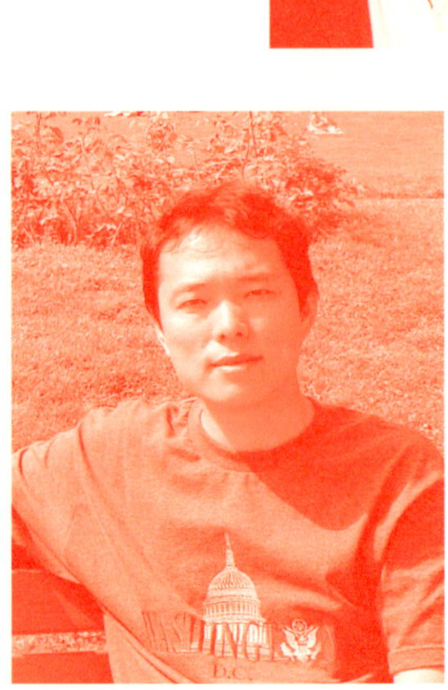
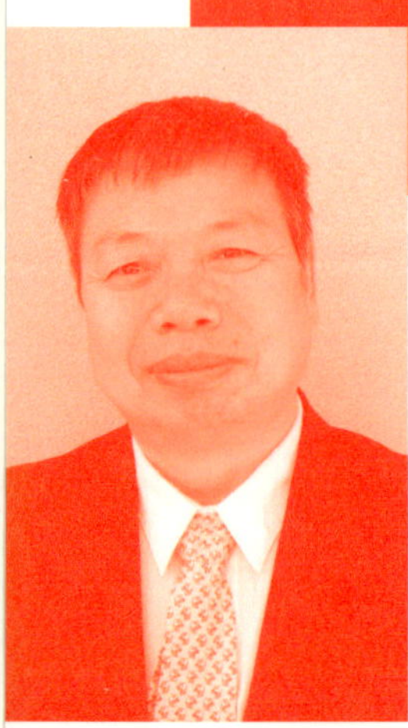
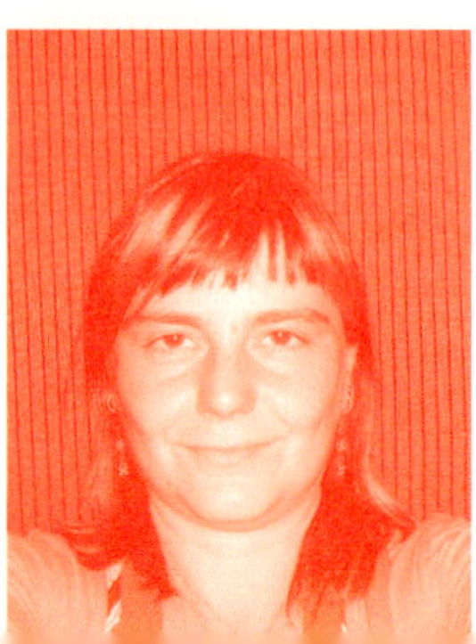

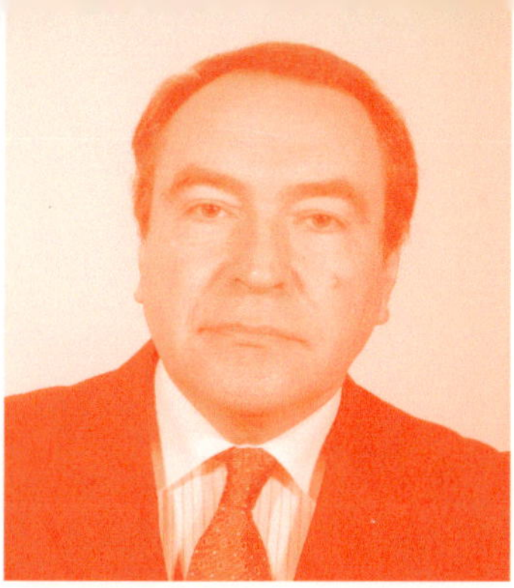
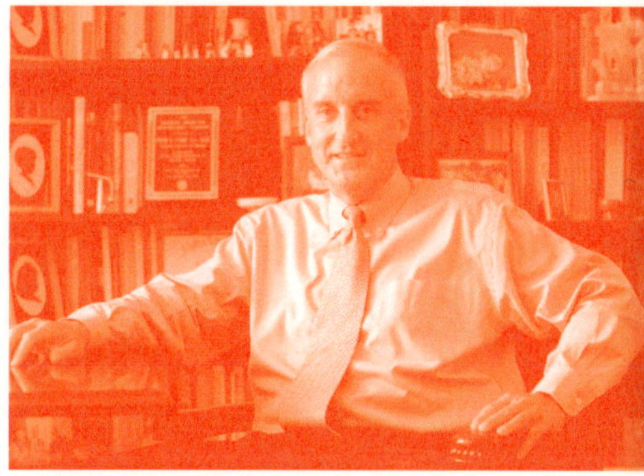
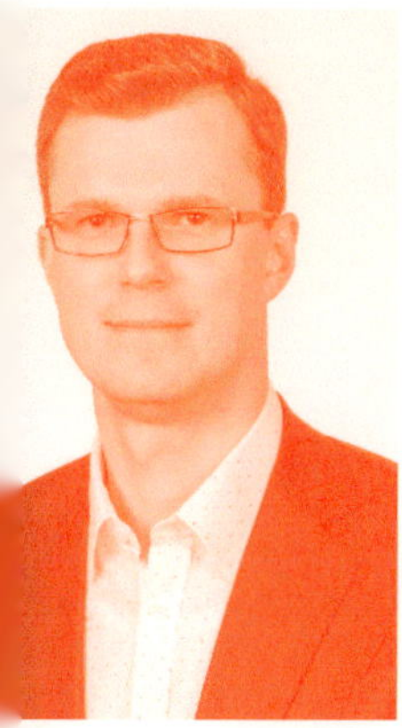
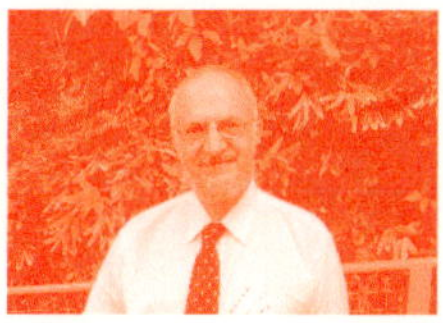
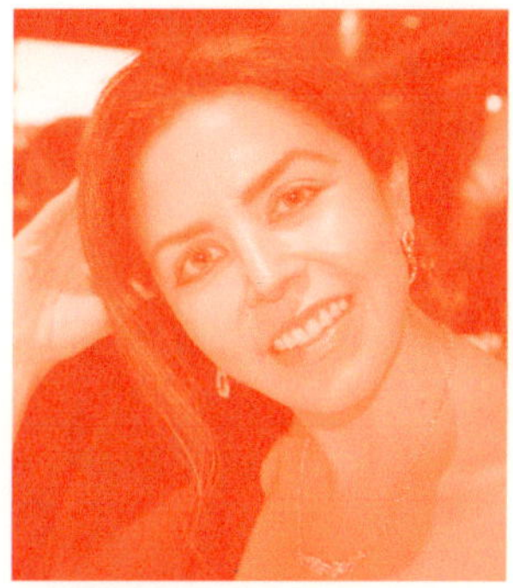

Supporting open minds since 2005

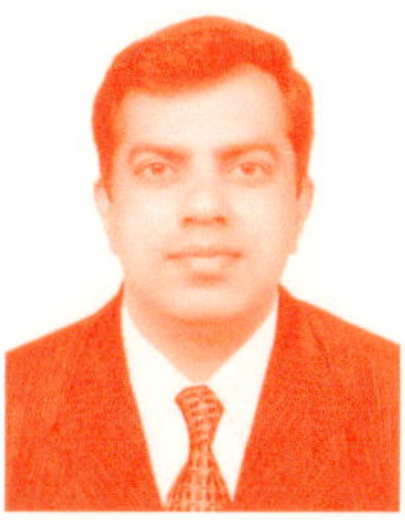
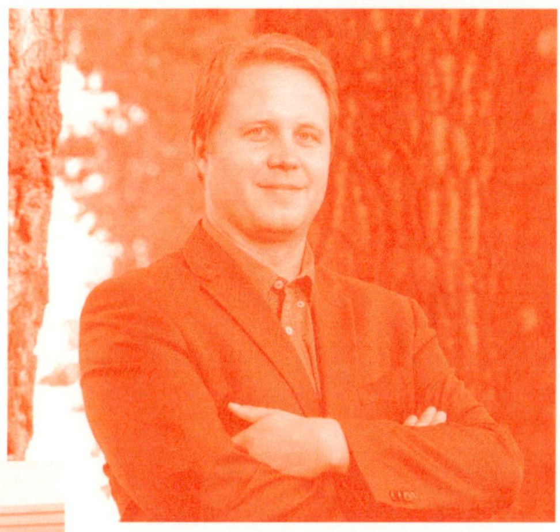
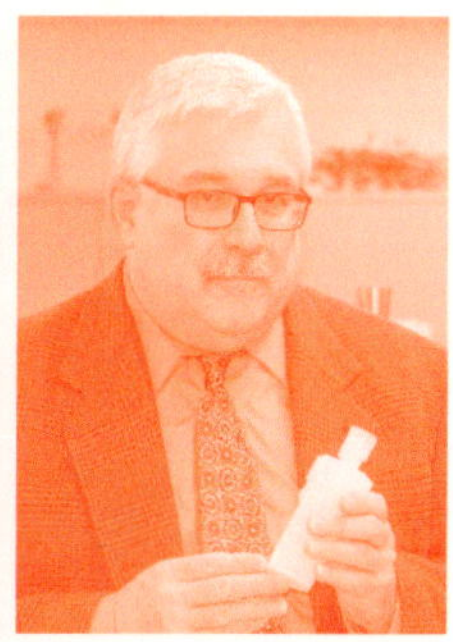
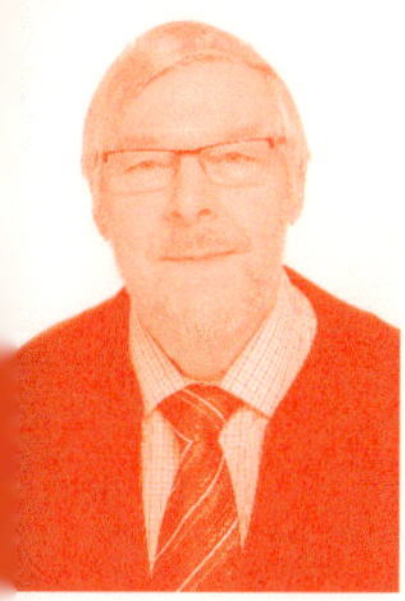
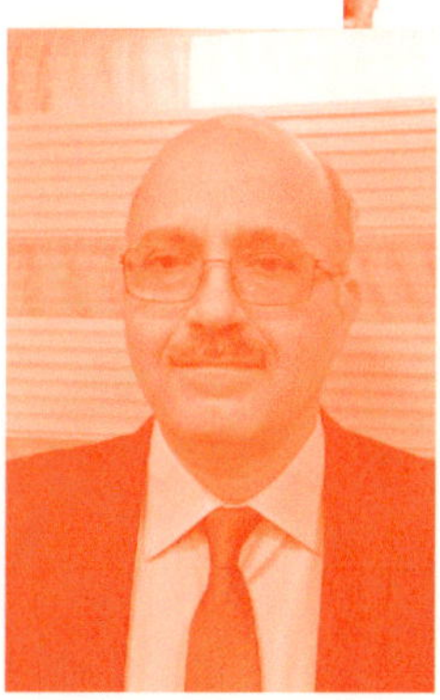
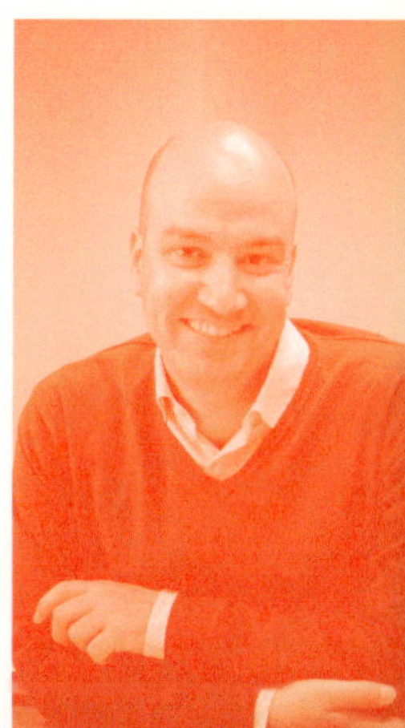
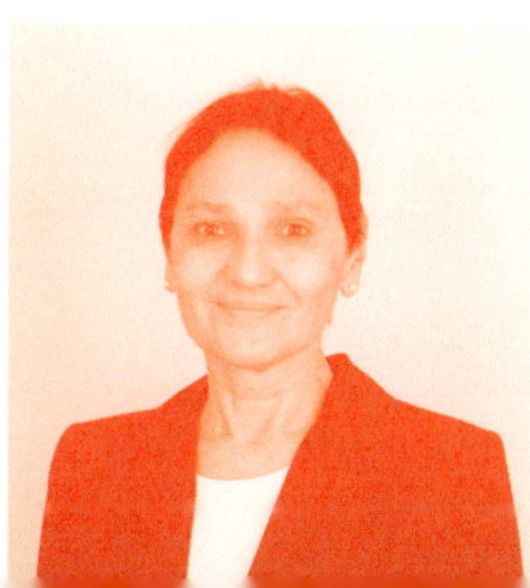

Current Concepts in Zika Research
http://dx.doi.org/10.5772/intechopen.82953
Edited by Alfonso J. Rodriguez-Morales

Contributors
Pablo Manrique-Saide, Silvina Contreras-Capetillo, Norma Pavia-Ruz, Yamila Romer, Nina Valadez-González, Hector Gomez-Dantés, Gonzalo Vazquez-Prokopec, Dayron Fernando Martinez-Pulgarin, Carlos Miguel Córdoba Ortega, Fabio Daniel Padilla-Pantoja, Diana Dimitrova, Thomas Harbo, Henning Andersen, Shannan Rossi, Rafael K Campos, Erin McDonald, Aaron Brault, Raafat Hammad Seroor Jadah, Alfonso J. Rodriguez-Morales, Carlos Andrés Rosero-Oviedo, D. Katterine Bonilla-Aldana, Jaime A. Cardona-Ospina, Wilmer Ernesto Villamil Gomez

First published in London, United Kingdom, 2021 by IntechOpen
IntechOpen is the global imprint of INTECHOPEN LIMITED, registered in England and Wales, registration number: 11086078, 5 Princes Gate Court, London, SW7 2QJ, United Kingdom
Printed in Croatia

British Library Cataloguing-in-Publication Data
A catalogue record for this book is available from the British Library

Additional hard and PDF copies can be obtained from orders@intechopen.com

Current Concepts in Zika Research
Edited by Alfonso J. Rodriguez-Morales
p. cm.
Print ISBN 978-1-83880-875-4
Online ISBN 978-1-83880-876-1
eBook (PDF) ISBN 978-1-83880-877-8

For EU product safety concerns:
IN TECH d.o.o., Prolaz Marije Krucifikse Kozulić 3, 51000 Rijeka, Croatia, info@intechopen.com or visit our website at intechopen.com.

Meet the editor

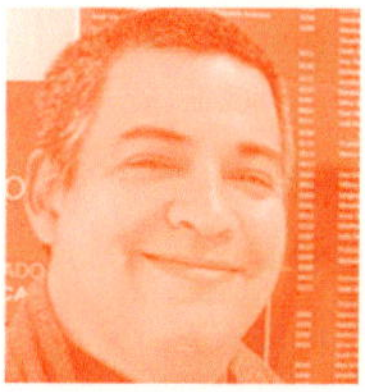

Dr. Alfonso J. Rodriguez-Morales received his Medical Doctor (MD) degree from the Universidad Central de Venezuela, Caracas, and his Master of Sciences in Protozoology/Parasitology (MSc) from the Universidad de Los Andes, Trujillo, Venezuela. He received his Diploma in Tropical Medicine & Hygiene (DT-M&H) from the Universidad Peruana Cayetano Heredia, Lima, Peru, and the University of Alabama at Birmingham, Birmingham, Alabama, USA. He is a Fellow of the Royal Society for Tropical Medicine & Hygiene (FRSTMH), London, United Kingdom; a Fellow of the Faculty of Travel Medicine (FFTM) of the Royal College of Physicians and Surgeons of Glasgow (RCPSG), Glasgow, Scotland, United Kingdom; and a Fellow of the American College of Epidemiology (FACE), USA. He is a Doctor of Sciences honoris causa (HonDSc) from the Universidad Privada Franz Tamayo (UniFranz), Cochabamba, Bolivia. Prof. Rodriguez-Morales is the President of the Travel Medicine Committee, Pan American Infectious Diseases Association, and the Vicepresident of the Colombian Infectious Diseases Association (2019-2021). He is a Member of the Council (2020-2026) of the International Society for Infectious Diseases (ISID). He is a Senior Researcher of Colciencias (2015-2021), and a Professor at the Universidad Tecnológica de Pereira and Fundación Universitaria Autónoma de las Américas, Pereira, Risaralda, Colombia. He is also a Visiting Professor at multiple national and international universities (H index=35, 508 articles at Scopus, 462 at PubMed and 441 at Web of Sciences).

Contents

Preface

Before 2013, yellow fever and dengue were the main arboviruses of concern in the Latin American region. However, after December of that year, chikungunya arrived in the region, and a couple of years later Zika virus (ZIKV) [1–16]. Zika is another virus transmitted by vectors (arboviruses) affecting not only people living in the tropics, but also travelers and migrating populations [17–20]. Zika has impacted significantly on the health of the Americas, especially in Central and South America, due to the large number of cases of Guillain-Barré Syndrome that have been reported in the association, as well, especially due to microcephaly and the Congenital Zika Syndrome, which was the reason for it to be declared on February 2016 as a Public Health Emergency of International Concern (PHEIC) by the World Health Organization (WHO) [1–16].

Keeping these issues in mind, this book includes different topics regarding research and clinical topics related to Zika virus research in the last five years in the Americas as well as in the World. This book has been organized in three major sections: Epidemiology; Clinical Aspects; and Zika and Guillain-Barré Syndrome.

Commissioning of this book by IntechOpen editorial has been related in part to my long commitment to vector-borne, zoonotic, and neglected tropical diseases, being involved as Co-Chair of the Working Group on Zoonoses of the International Society for Chemotherapy (WGZ-ISC), as well as in Colombia at the Committee on Tropical Medicine, Zoonoses and Travel Medicine of the Colombian Association of Infectious Diseases (Asociación Colombiana de Infectología, ACIN) and more recently important, as the Chair of the Colombian Collaborative Network of Research on Zika (Red Colombiana de Colaboración en Zika) (RECOLZIKA), since January 2016. RECOLZIKA has contributed to multiple aspects of the research on Zika in Colombia and other countries in Latin America, including about the Congenital Zika Syndrome as well as on the Guillain-Barré, among other clinical consequences of this arboviral disease (more than 50 papers in journals indexed on Scopus, Web of Sciences and PubMed, among other databases).

I have been involved in tropical diseases for the last two decades, including leishmaniasis, Chagas disease, as well as dengue, and since 2014, chikungunya and emerging arboviruses, such as Zika and Mayaro. After moving from Venezuela to Colombia in 2011, I have been involved in research of tropical diseases in Risaralda, such as leishmaniasis (still prevalent in the area), where we still keep working on this important neglected condition. Part of all this is a clear reflection of the work at the Research Group Infection Public Health and Infection (classified A1 by Colciencias) of the Faculty of Health Sciences of the Universidad Tecnológica de Pereira, directed by Dr. Guillermo Javier Lagos-Grisales, not just a partner, a colleague and mainly a friend, an extreme believer in our work in vector-borne and zoonotic diseases. But, I must recognize also the beginning of a significant collaboration after a meeting in Cartagena in 2013, during the Colombian Congress of Infectious Diseases, where I met Dr. Wilmer Ernesto Villamil-Gómez, from Sincelejo, Sucre, Colombia, also part of the former Committee of Zoonoses and Hemorrhagic Fevers of the Colombian Association of Infectious Diseases (Asociación Colombiana de Infectología, ACIN) (now called Committee of Zoonoses and Tropical Medicine), who became since that year my most important collaborator on arboviruses, including Zika. In addition to that, since 2002 I have been involved in tropical medicine and travel medicine, participating in multiple studies on Chagas disease, leishmaniasis, and other tropical diseases. Currently in Colombia, we continue studying most of them, including now their assessment in internally displaced populations.

Following the same philosophy as we had on my eight previous books with IntechOpen, Current Topics in Tropical Medicine [21], Current Topics in Public Health [22], Current Topics in Echinococcosis [23], Current Topics in Chikungunya [24], Current Topics in Malaria [25], Current Topics in Giardiasis [26], Current Topics in Zika [27], Current Topics in Tropical Emerging Infectious Diseases and Travel Medicine [28], Current Topics in Neglected Tropical Diseases [29], this books does not intend to be an exhaustive compilation and this first edition has included not just multiple different topics but also wide geographical participation from many countries of different regions of the world. In a previous book, Current Topics in Zika [27], many related topics have been developed. This updated book with complementary topics includes new contributors and perspectives. Its online availability through the website of IntechOpen, as well the possibility to upload the complete book or their chapters on personal websites and institution repositories, allows it to reach a wide audience. Continuing on the series of "Current Topics" books, we are planning to develop in the future other projects such as "Current Topics in Zoonoses", "Current Topics in Virology", "Current Topics in COVID-19".

I would like to give a very special thanks to IntechOpen, and particularly to Josip Knapic, for the opportunity to edit this interesting and important book, as well for his constant support.

I want to take the appropriate time and space, as I used to do, to dedicate this book to my beloved family (Aurora, Alfonso José, Alejandro and Andrea, the neurologist). Katterine, my fiancé, is making every day more and more special my life, I love her more than anything and I am happy to have her existence in my life. I love you.

Also, to my friends and my undergraduate and postgraduate students of health sciences in Colombia, Venezuela and around Latin America. Also is time to say thanks to my colleagues at the Working Group on Zoonoses, International Society for Chemotherapy and the Committee on Zoonoses, Tropical Medicine and Travel Medicine (formerly on Zoonoses and Haemorrhagic Fevers) of the Colombian Infectious Diseases Society (ACIN) and a large list of members of RECOLZIKA (www.RECOLZIKA.org). Special thanks again to my friend and colleague Dr. Guillermo J. Lagos-Grisales, MD, MPH. Members of our research group and incubator consist of young and enthusiastic medical students and some veterinary medical students as well as young medical doctors, who are pursuing significant improvements in the understanding of the epidemiology of zoonotic, vector-borne, parasitic and in general, infectious diseases, in our country with international projection. The year 2019 has been a great year, very productive for this recognized group, which was classified in 2017 by the national agency of science, Colciencias, in the highest rank "A1", and then again in 2019 recognized with that rank, which is positioning as a leader in infectious diseases epidemiology research in the coffee-triangle region and in the country. The idea of this book begun in 2019, but in 2020 we faced the COVID-19 pandemic that certainly impacted multiple life processes including the development of this book, but certainly is a new pathogen we should also face, and indeed we also created a network for research and collaboration on this, LANCOVID (www.LANCOVID.org).

Finally, I hope our readers enjoy this publication as much as I did reading the chapters of Current Concepts in Zika Research.

Alfonso J. Rodriguez-Morales MD, MSc, DTM&H, FRSTMH(Lon), FFTM RCPS(Glasg), FACE, HonDSc.
Professor,
Editor, Current Concepts in Zika Research,
Senior Researcher, Public Health and Infection Research Group,
Faculty of Health Sciences,
Universidad Tecnológica de Pereira,
Pereira, Risaralda, Colombia

Senior Researcher, Grupo de Investigación Biomedicina,
Faculty of Medicine,
Fundación Universitaria Autónoma de las Américas,
Pereira, Risaralda, Colombia

Chair, Colombian Network of Research in Zika (RECOLZIKA),
Pereira, Risaralda, Colombia

Chair, Latin American Network of Coronavirus Disease 2019 Research (LANCOVID),
Pereira, Risaralda, Colombia

Co-Chair, Working Group on Zoonoses,
International Society for Chemotherapy (ISC),
Pereira, Risaralda, Colombia

Vicepresident, Colombian Association of Infectious Diseases (ACIN),
Pereira, Risaralda, Colombia

Member of the Committee on Tropical Medicine,
Zoonoses and Travel Medicine, ACIN,
Pereira, Risaralda, Colombia

President, Committee on Travel Medicine,
Pan-American Association of Infectious Diseases,
Panama City, Panama

References

[1] Rodriguez-Morales AJ, Bandeira AC, Franco-Paredes C. The expanding spectrum of modes of transmission of Zika virus: a global concern. Ann Clin Microbiol Antimicrob. 2016 Mar 3; 15:13. http://dx.doi.org/10.1186/s12941-016-0128-2

[2] Rodriguez-Morales AJ, Cardona-Ospina JA, Ramirez-Jaramillo V, Gaviria JA, González-Moreno GM, Castrillón-Spitia JD, López-Villegas A, Morales-Jiménez E, Ramírez-Zapata V, Rueda-Merchán GE, Trujillo AM, Tabares-Villa FA, Henao-SanMartin V, Murillo-Garcia DR, Herrera-Soto JA, Buitrago-Cañas ML, Collins MH, Sepúlveda-Arias JC, Londoño JJ, Bedoya-Rendón HD, Cárdenas-Pérez JJ, Olaya SX, Lagos-Grisales GJ. Diagnosis and outcomes of pregnant women with Zika virus infection in two municipalities of Risaralda, Colombia: Second report of the ZIKERNCOL study. Travel Med Infect Dis 2018 Sep-Oct; 25(10):20-25

[3] Rodríguez-Morales AJ, Bonilla-Aldana DK, Bonilla-Aldana JL, Arteaga-Livias K, Pecho-Silva S, Escalera-Antezana JP. Role of Zika virus infection in cases and outbreaks of Guillain-Barré syndrome in Latin America: pooling the prevalence of studies. Travel Med Infect Dis 2021 Epub Ahead Nov 1; https://www.sciencedirect.com/science/article/abs/pii/S1477893920304014

[4] Alvarado-Socarras JL, Idrovo AJ, Contreras-García GA, Rodriguez-Morales AJ, Audcent TA, Mogollon-Mendoza AC, Paniz-Mondolfi A. Congenital microcephaly: A diagnostic challenge during Zika epidemics. Travel Med Infect Dis 2018 May-Jun; 23(3):14-20.

[5] Bonilla-Aldana DK, Bonilla-Aldana JL, García-Bustos JJ, Lozada CO, Rodríguez-Morales AJ. Geographical Trends of Chikungunya and Zika in the Colombian Amazonian Gateway Department, Caqueta, 2015-2018 – Implications for Public Health and Travel Medicine. Travel Med Infect Dis 2020 May-Jun; 35:101481.

[6] Chowdhury FR, Ibrahim QSU, Bari S, Alam MMJ, Dunachie SJ, Rodriguez-Morales AJ, Patwary I. The Association between Temperature, Rainfall and Humidity with Common Climate-sensitive infectious Diseases in Bangladesh. PLoS One 2018; 13(6):e0199579. doi 10.1371/ journal.pone.0199579

[7] Quintero-Herrera LL, Ramírez-Jaramillo V, Bernal-Gutiérrez S, Cárdenas-Giraldo EV, Guerrero-Matituy EA, Molina-Delgado AH, Montoya-Arias CP, Rico-Gallego JA, Herrera-Giraldo AC, Botero-Franco S, Rodríguez-Morales AJ. Potential impact of climatic variability on the epidemiology of Dengue in Risaralda, Colombia, 2010-2011. J Infect Public Health 2015 May-June; 8(3):291-297.

[8] Escobedo AA, Almirall P, Rumbaut R, Rodríguez-Morales AJ. Potential impact of macroclimatic variability on the epidemiology of Giardiasis in three provinces of Cuba, 2010-2012. J Infect Public Health 2015 Jan-Feb; 8(1):80-89.

[9] Mattar S, Morales V, Cassab A, Rodríguez-Morales AJ. Effect of Climate Variables on Dengue Incidence in a Tropical Caribbean Municipality of Colombia, Cerete, 2003-2008. Int J Infect Dis 2013 May; 17(5):e358-e359.

[10] Rodriguez-Morales AJ. Climate Change, Climate Variability and Brucellosis. Recent Pat Antiinfect Drug Discov 2013; 8(1):4-12.

[11] Von A, Zaragoza E, Jones D, Rodríguez-Morales AJ, Franco-Paredes C. New insights into Chagas

Disease: a neglected disease in Latin America. J Infect Dev Ctries 2007 Oct; 1(2):99-111.

[12] Franco-Paredes C, Jones D, Rodriguez-Morales AJ, Santos-Preciado JI. Commentary: Improving the health of neglected populations in Latin America. BMC Public Health 2007 Jan 23;7:11.

[13] Rodriguez-Morales AJ, Bolívar-Mejía A, Alarcón-Olave C, Calvo-Betancourt LS. Plasmodium vivax Malaria in Latin America. In: C. Franco-Paredes, J.I. Santos-Preciado (eds.). Neglected Tropical Diseases – Latin America and the Caribbean, Neglected Tropical Diseases. Springer-Verlag Wien, 2015. doi: 10.1007/978-3-7091-1422-3_5. Pages 23. ISBN 978-3-7091-1421-6. Pp: 89-111.

[14] Franco-Paredes C and Rodríguez-Morales AJ. Awakening Hippocrates: A Primer on Health, Poverty, and Global Service. JAMA 2006 Aug 2; 296(5): 591.

[15] Quintero K, Durán C, Duri D, Medina F, Garcia J, Hidalgo G, Nakal S, Echeverria-Ortega M, Albano C, Nino Incani R, Cortez J, Jiménez S, Díaz M, Maldonado C, Matute F, Rodriguez-Morales AJ. Household social determinants of ascariasis and trichuriasis in North Central Venezuela. International Health 2012 Jun; 4(2): 103-110.

[16] Franco-Paredes C, Rodriguez-Morales AJ. Unsolved matters in leprosy: a descriptive review and call for further research. Ann Clin Microbiol Antimicrob. 2016 May 21; 15:33. http://ann-clinmicrob.biomedcentral.com/articles/10.1186/s12941-016-0149-x

[17] Musso D, Rodriguez-Morales AJ, Levi JE, Cao-Lormeau VM, Gubler DJ. Unexpected outbreaks of arbovirus infections: Lessons Learned from the Pacific and Tropical America. Lancet Infect Dis 2018 Nov; 18(11):e355-e361.

[18] Pezzi L, Reusken CB, Weaver SC, Drexler JF, Busch M, LaBeaud D, Diamond MS, Vasilakis N, Drebot MA, Siqueira AM, Ribeiro GS, Kohl A, Lecuit M, Ng LFP, Gallian P, de Lamballerie X, on behalf of GloPID-R Chikungunya, O'nyong-nyong and Mayaro virus Working Group, Boyer S, Brasil P, Diallo M, Failloux AB, Jaenisch T, Lourenço-de-Oliveira R, Neyts J, Rios M, Rodriguez-Morales AJ, Rosa-Freitas MG, Sall A, Simmons G, Simon F, Vega Rua A. GloPID-R report on Chikungunya, O'nyong-nyong and Mayaro virus, part I: Biological diagnostics. Antiviral Research 2019 Jun; 166:66-81.

[19] Pezzi L, LaBeaud D, Reusken CB, Drexler JF, Vasilakis N, Diallo M, Simon F, Jaenisch T, Gallian P, Sall A, Failloux AB, Weaver SC, Lamballerie X, on behalf of GloPID-R Chikungunya, O'nyong-nyong and Mayaro virus Working Group, de Boyer S, Brasil P, Busch M, Diamond MS, Drebot MA, Kohl A, Lecuit M, Lourenço-de-Oliveira R, Neyts J, Ng LFP, Ribeiro GS, Rios M, Rodriguez-Morales AJ, Rosa-Freitas MG, Simmons G, Siqueira AM, Vega Rua A. GloPID-R report on Chikungunya, O'nyong-nyong and Mayaro virus, part II: Epidemiological distribution of O'nyong-nyong virus. Antiviral Research 2019 Epub Ahead Sep 20 https://www.sciencedirect.com/science/article/pii/S0166354219305121

[20] Pezzi L, Rodriguez-Morales AJ, Reusken CB, Ribeiro GS, LaBeaud D, Lourenço-de-Oliveira R, Brasil P, Lecuit M, Failloux AB, Gallian P, Jaenisch T, Simon F, Siqueira AM, Rosa-Freitas MG, Vega Rua A, Weaver SC, Drexler JF, Vasilakis N, Lamballerie X, on behalf of GloPID-R Chikungunya, O'nyong-nyong and Mayaro virus Working Group. GloPID-R report on Chikungunya, O'nyong-nyong and Mayaro virus, part III: Epidemiological distribution of Mayaro virus. Antiviral Research 2019 Epub Ahead Sep 20 https://www.sciencedirect.com/science/article/pii/S0166354219305133

[21] Rodriguez-Morales AJ. (Editor). Current Topics in Tropical Medicine. ISBN 978-953-51-0274-8. InTech, Croatia, March 2012. Available at: http://www.intechopen.com/books/current-topics-in-tropical-medicine

[22] Rodriguez-Morales AJ. (Editor). Current Topics in Public Health. ISBN 978-953-51-1121-4. InTech, Croatia, May 2013. Available at: http://www.intechopen.com/books/current-topics-in-public-health

[23] Rodriguez-Morales AJ. (Editor). Current Topics in Echinococcosis. ISBN 978-953-51-2159-6. InTech, Croatia, September 2015. http://www.intechopen.com/books/current-topics-in-echinococcosis

[24] Rodriguez-Morales AJ. (Editor). Current Topics in Chikungunya. ISBN 978-953-51-2595-2. InTech, Croatia, August 2016. http://www.intechopen.com/books/current-topics-in-chikungunya

[25] Rodriguez-Morales AJ. (Editor). Current Topics in Malaria. ISBN 978-953-51-2790-1. InTech, Croatia, November 2016. http://www.intechopen.com/books/current-topics-in-malaria

[26] Rodriguez-Morales AJ. (Editor). Current Topics in Giardiasis. ISBN 978-953-51-5260-6. InTech, Croatia, December 2017. http://www.intechopen.com/books/current-topics-in-giardiasis

[27] Rodriguez-Morales AJ. (Editor). Current Topics in Zika. ISBN 978-1-78923-271-4. InTech, United Kingdom, June 2018. https://www.intechopen.com/books/current-topics-in-zika

[28] Rodriguez-Morales AJ. (Editor). Current Topics in Tropical Emerging Diseases and Travel Medicine. ISBN 978-1-78984-824-3. InTech, United Kingdom, December 2018. https://www.intechopen.com/books/current-topics-in-tropical-emerging-diseases-and-travel-medicine

[29] Rodriguez-Morales AJ. (Editor). Current Topics in Neglected Tropical Diseases. ISBN 978-1-78923-890-7. InTech, United Kingdom, December 2019. Available at: https://www.intechopen.com/books/current-topics-in-neglected-tropical-diseases

Section 1

Epidemiology

Chapter 1

Introductory Chapter: Zika 2015-2020 - Knowledge and Experience in the Americas

Carlos Andrés Rosero-Oviedo, D. Katterine Bonilla-Aldana, Jaime A. Cardona-Ospina, Wilmer E. Villamil-Gómez and Alfonso J. Rodriguez-Morales

1. Introduction

Zika virus is an arbovirus that was discovered many decades ago but remains fundamentally silent until a couple of decades ago. Nevertheless, only when arrived in the Americas, was able to cause significant epidemics and new clinical consequences, including microcephaly and the Guillain-Barré syndrome, among others. In this chapter, we introduce general concepts and our position regard the relevance of Zika and their knowledge and experience in the Americas over the last years, 2015–2020.

2. Fundamental aspects of Zika virus and Zika disease

The Zika virus (ZIKV) was first isolated in Uganda in 1947 and was confined for almost 60 years in Africa and Asia. Later, in 2007, the Yap outbreak allowed its spread to French Polynesia and other Pacific islands in 2013–2015, finally reaching the Americas in 2015 and being declared a Public Health Emergency of International Importance in 2016. Currently, no area is reporting Zika outbreaks; however, its circulation through sporadic cases remains a global threat. The discovery of ZIKV and many other arboviruses was the result of research conducted within the Rockefeller Foundation-sponsored yellow fever research programs [1]. The current East African Virus Research Institute (Entebbe, Uganda), was a focal point for research on pathogenic viruses. In April 1947, in an attempt to map the spread of yellow fever, the temperature of Rhesus monkeys, of the Asian species (*Macaca mulatta*), used in six sentinel platforms in the Zika forest in Entebbe, Uganda, was measured periodically [2]. On April 18, 1947, the temperature of one of these monkeys, Rhesus 766, was reported to be 39.7°C and the next day 40°C, so it was taken to the Entebbe laboratory where it was kept under observation for 30 days, with no evidence of other symptoms. On the third day of fever, a blood sample was taken that would subsequently allow the isolation of what was called ZIKV (strain 766). In the same report, the first isolation of ZIKV is described in 86 Aedes africanus mosquitoes trapped on a tree platform in the Zika forest in January 1948 [2]. Interestingly, although there was no evidence that ZIKV caused disease among Ugandan residents, the prevalence of antibodies to ZIKV was 9.5–20%, suggesting that the virus was already circulating in the human population (or was a consequence of cross-reactivity with other flaviviruses) [3]. A more detailed description of the origins of ZIKV is presented elsewhere [4]. Although the initial isolation and characterisation of ZIKV in Uganda's Zika forest are unquestionable, there is some controversy as to which report described the first human ZIKV infection [5]. Several authors suggest that the first isolation in humans was in 1954, and it was a 10-year-old African girl with fever and headache associated with a malaria co-infection [6]. Cross-neutralisation tests with convalescent sera from monkeys infected with different viruses indicated that only ZIKV-infected serum neutralised the virus from the patient's serum, strongly suggesting ZIKV infection. However, a later published report indicated that the virus isolated in West Africa was more closely related to the Sponweni virus, and not to the Zika virus [7]. Ten years later, in 1964, a report is published of a worker at the East African Virus Research Institute in Entebbe who became infected with ZIKV while working on a series of new ZIKV strains, and his clinical presentation was characterised headache, diffuse pink maculopapular rash, myalgia, fever, and general malaise [8]. Interestingly, the author of the report is the same infected patient.

Outside of Africa, ZIKV was first isolated in 1969, in one of 58 groups of 1,277 *Aedes aegypti* mosquitoes collected from cities and towns on the Malay Peninsula (now Malaysia, Asia) [9]. Then, in 1977 in Indonesia (Asia), human infections of ZIKV infection were described, which were clinically characterised by high fever, malaise, stomach pain, dizziness and anorexia [10]. Notably, apart from direct evidence on ZIKV circulation from previously described human isolates and cases of infection, serological studies conducted in the 1950s suggest that ZIKV had a widespread distribution in both Africa (East, Central, West and South) as in several Asian countries [11]. However, the interpretation of serological results should be made with caution because the cross-reactions were not well characterised at that time [12]. From the first report of ZIKV infection in humans in 1954 (or 1964) through the early 2000s, only a few isolated cases of ZIKV infection disease have been documented. However, the outbreak in Yap State "initiates" the events that would make ZIKV a potential pandemic threat and are briefly described in **Figure 1**. Other publications describe these milestones in more detail [13–26].

The ZIKV is a member of the Flaviviridae family of viruses, which includes small viruses with a positive single-stranded RNA genome (9000–13000 bases) and which in turn is composed of 4 genera (Flavivirus, Hepacivirus [hepatitis C virus], Pegivirus and Pestivirus) [27]. Although transmission through mosquito bites is the

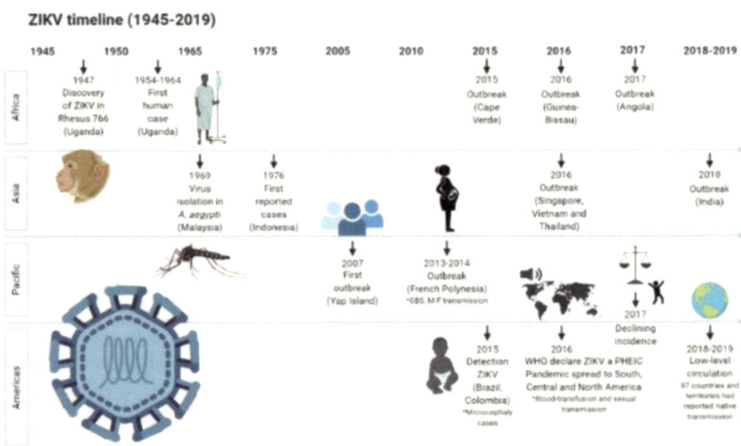

Figure 1.
*Chronology of ZIKV infection and reported cases. *ZIKV = Zika virus; GBS = Guillain-Barré syndrome; M-F = Maternal-fetal; PHEIC = Public Health Emergency of International Concern.*

primary mechanism for the spread of ZIKV, other routes of transmission have been proposed that contribute to the epidemic.

Vector transmission: Transmission through the bite of infected mosquitoes is the primary mechanism for the spread of ZIKV. The *Aedes aegypti* mosquito is the primary vector for urban transmission of ZIKV throughout the world. At the same time, other Aedes species can act as vectors for ZIKV in specific environments where its abundance is essential (e.g. *A. albopictus* that lives in temperate regions) [29]. Aedes mosquitoes can also transmit dengue and chikungunya viruses.

Non-vector transmission: Non-vector transmission events have been reported including maternal-fetal transmission, sexual transmission, transmission associated with transfusion of blood products or organ transplantation, and laboratory exposure [30, 31].

3. Clinical features

Possibly the first clinical description of a patient with ZIKV was reported in 1956 [32]. It was a 34-year-old European volunteer who was inoculated subcutaneously with a strain of ZIKV from Nigeria. After an incubation period of 82 hours, he developed a frontal headache associated with mild and short-term fever. On the afternoon of the fifth day, the headache, fever, and malaise increased in severity. It was accompanied by nausea and vertigo (which was attributed to a histamine reaction that responded to a small dose of aspirin). By the seventh day, the patient had fully recovered [32]. The percentage of asymptomatic ZIKV infections is estimated to be 50–80% [16, 33]. Data obtained from the Yap Island seroprevalence study showed that only 19% of those infected had symptoms attributable to ZIKV [34]. However, the retrospective seroprevalence study in French Polynesia showed that, among ZIKV seropositive patients, the percentage of symptomatic infections was 47% in adults [35]. That suggests that the virus strain could influence the proportion of symptomatic ZIKV infections.

For symptomatic infections, the incubation period varies from 3 to 14 days [36], and in most cases, the disease is self-limited [37]. It generally manifests as an itchy rash, mild fever, fatigue, myalgia/arthralgia, conjunctivitis, and headache, with an average duration of 1 week [37, 38]. The clinical characteristics appear to be similar in all age groups, regardless of sex and gestational status. Serious illness requiring hospitalisation is rare [9–48]. As observed, especially in some countries of Latin America, comorbidities would complicated cases [21–48].

The frequency of complications related to ZIKV infection appears to be low, but when they do occur, they are severe and can be fatal [39]. The most commonly reported complications to include complications associated with ZIKV infection during pregnancy such as congenital ZIKV syndrome (CZS), microcephaly, congenital malformations or abnormalities, brain abnormalities (e.g., delayed brain growth), eye disorders, pregnancy, fetal or perinatal death, hearing disorders, cardiovascular damage, neurological complications, intrauterine growth restriction, amniotic fluid abnormalities and epilepsy; neurological complications in adults, such as Guillain-Barré syndrome (https://www.who.int/csr/disease/zika/case-definition/en/); and finally death associated with ZIKV infection [40–49].

4. Diagnosis

Because the clinical manifestations of acute ZIKV infection are nonspecific, the definitive diagnosis is made by molecular and serological methods [43]. However, clinical and epidemiological criteria justify screening tests.

4.1 Clinical

For ZIKV disease, the clinical criteria for the definition of a suspected case according to the Centers for Disease Control and Prevention (CDC, 2016) corresponds to a person with one or more of the following (not explained by another aetiology) [15–44]:

Suspected case:

- Clinically compatible disease including acute onset of fever (measured or reported), maculopapular rash, arthralgia or conjunctivitis; or
- Guillain-Barré syndrome or other neurological manifestations; or
- Complications of pregnancy (e.g., loss of a fetus, fetus or newborn with congenital microcephaly, congenital intracranial calcifications, structural abnormalities of the brain or eyes, or structural abnormalities related to the central nervous system).

Epidemiological link criteria:

- Recent residence or travel to areas with known ZIKV transmission, sexual contact with a confirmed or probable case within the transmission risk window (2 weeks).
- Receipt of blood, blood products or organ or tissue transplantation within 30 days after the onset of symptoms.
- Association in time and place with a confirmed or probable case; and
- Probable vector exposure in an area with suitable ecological and seasonal conditions for possible local vector transmission.

*An online resource is available through the CDC website (https://wwwnc.cdc.gov/travel/page/zika-information) to recognise areas with reported cases of ZIKV infection.

4.2 Laboratory

The diagnostic approach to ZIKV infection may vary depending on the resources available. For patients with suspected ZIKV disease, molecular detection of ZIKV RNA (e.g. nucleic acid amplification tests or NAAT [by RT-PCR]) is the preferred diagnostic method because they can provide confirmed evidence of infection and distinguish the specific virus [45, 46]. However, nucleic acid tests only show the presence of ZIKV RNA but do not necessarily indicate the presence of infectious viruses. On the other hand, serological tests (e.g. IgM antibodies [employing an immunosorbent assay linked to IgM antibody capture enzymes or MAC-ELISA]) or IgG [by plaque reduction neutralisation test or PRNT] against ZIKV are They are used mainly in patients who present after the viral nucleic acid is no longer detectable [20–48], despite the number of false-positive results due to cross-reactivity with other flaviviruses.

The algorithm for recommendations and the interpretation of the results of the dengue virus and ZIKV diagnostic tests are described in **Figure 2**.

4.2.1 Pregnant women

Pregnant women with a clinically compatible disease and possible exposure to ZIKV or dengue virus should be evaluated as soon as possible (**Figure 3**). Evaluation for ZIKV and dengue infection is performed by performing NAAT and IgM antibody testing on serum sample and NAAT on a urine sample. NAATs can be performed on

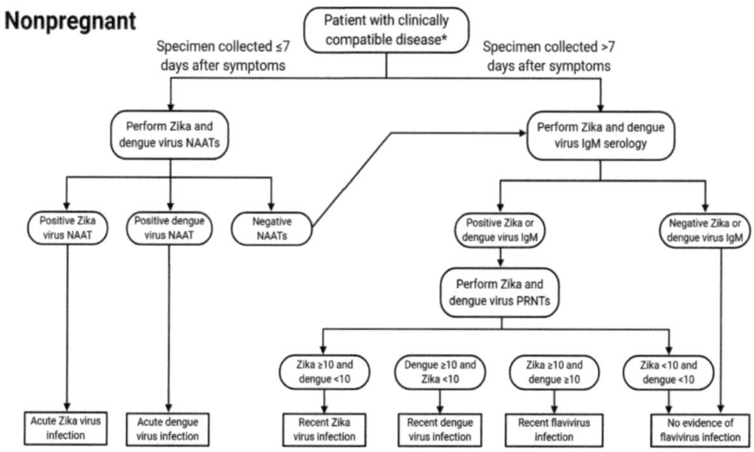

NAAT = nucleic acid amplification test; PRNT = plaque reduction neutralization test. Selection of samples and tests: Dengue virus and ZIKV NAATs, IgM antibody tests and PRNTs must be performed on serum. Some NAATs can also be performed on plasma, whole blood, cerebrospinal fluid, or urine, and some antibody tests can be performed on plasma, whole blood, or cerebrospinal fluid. Laboratories may choose to test for Dengue virus and ZIKV IgM and NAAT antibodies simultaneously rather than sequentially, or to test Dengue virus nonstructural protein one rather than Dengue virus NAAT. Indications for repeat testing: If the patient's disease is of epidemiological or clinical significance (e.g., the first case of local transmission in the area, a new mode of transmission, or unusual clinical syndrome), repeat a positive NAAT on fresh RNA extracted from the same sample. For indeterminate results of the IgM antibody test, repeat the IgM antibody test or perform a PRNT on the same sample. In areas where PRNT is not performed, report indeterminate results and request a second serum sample for IgM antibody testing. Interpretation of results: Dengue virus and ZIKV IgM antibodies can be detected in serum during the months after infection. The specific time of infection cannot be determined. Data on the epidemiology of viruses known to circulate at the site of exposure and clinical findings should be taken into account when interpreting the results of serological diagnostic tests.

Figure 2.
*Algorithm of recommendations for testing ZIKV and dengue virus for people with the clinically compatible disease and risk for infection with both viruses. *And risk for infection with both viruses. Adapted and modified from CDC.*

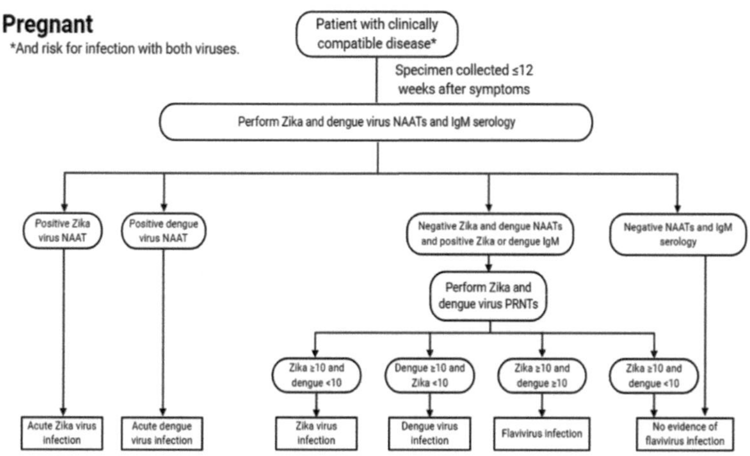

NAAT = nucleic acid amplification test; PRNT = plaque reduction neutralization test. * Selection of samples and tests: Dengue virus and ZIKV NAATs, IgM antibody tests and PRNTs must be performed on serum. Some NAATs can also be performed on plasma, whole blood, cerebrospinal fluid, or urine, and some antibody tests can be performed on plasma, whole blood, or cerebrospinal fluid. Dengue virus NAAT does not need to be performed on samples collected> 7 days after disease onset. Some laboratories may choose to test dengue virus nonstructural protein one instead of dengue virus NAAT. Indications for repeat testing: If the ZIKV NAAT is positive in a single sample, but the IgM antibody tests are negative, repeat the NAAT on freshly extracted RNA from the same sample. For indeterminate results of the IgM antibody test, repeat the IgM antibody test or perform a PRNT on the same sample. In areas where PRNT is not performed, report indeterminate results and request a second serum sample for IgM antibody testing. Interpretation of results: Dengue virus and ZIKV IgM antibodies can be detected in serum during the months after infection. The specific time of infection cannot be determined. Data on the epidemiology of viruses known to circulate at the site of exposure and clinical findings should be taken into account when interpreting the results of serological diagnostic tests.

Figure 3.
*Algorithm of recommendations for testing ZIKV and dengue virus for pregnant women with the clinically compatible disease and risk for infection with both viruses. *And risk for infection with both viruses. Adapted and modified from CDC.*

plasma, cerebrospinal fluid whole blood, or amniotic fluid; likewise, IgM antibody tests can be performed on plasma, whole blood, or cerebrospinal fluid. Specimens should be collected as soon as possible and within 12 weeks of the onset of symptoms. A positive NAAT result in any sample provides sufficient evidence of a recent infection. However, suppose the NAAT is only positive for ZIKV in a single sample, and the IgM antibody test is negative. In that case, the NAAT should be repeated with fresh RNA from the same sample to rule out false-positive results. If the NAAT is negative, but the IgM antibody test is positive, confirmatory PRNTs should be performed for dengue, ZIKV, and other flaviviruses endemic to the region (**Figure 3**).

For asymptomatic pregnant women without continued risk of possible Zika virus infection, routine screening for ZIKV infection is not recommended. However, the assessment must be considered in terms of risk and through a shared decision-making model. A more detailed review is described elsewhere [15–39].

The algorithm of recommendations and the interpretation of the results of the dengue virus and ZIKV diagnostic tests in pregnant women are described in **Figure 2**.

5. Classification of cases

The definition of suspected cases was previously described. According to the CDC [44], suspected cases should be classified into:

Probable case	Confirmed case
• Clinical criteria for ZIKV disease; and • Epidemiological link; and • Laboratory evidence of recent ZIKV or flavivirus infection by: o Positive test of IgM antibodies against ZIKV in serum or CSF; and o Positive neutralising antibody titers (e.g. PRNT) against ZIKV, dengue or other flaviviruses endemic to the region where the exposure occurred; or o Negative test for IgM antibodies against dengue virus, and no neutralising antibody tests were performed.	• Clinical criteria for ZIKV disease; and • Laboratory evidence of recent ZIKV infection by: o Detection of ZIKV by culture, viral antigen or viral RNA in serum, CSF, tissue or another sample (e.g. amniotic fluid, urine, semen, saliva); or o Positive serum or CSF IgM antibody test against ZIKV with positive ZIKV neutralising antibody titers (≥10) and negative neutralising antibody titers against dengue or other endemic flaviviruses in the region of exposure.

** The criteria for WHO/PAHO are similar (www.paho.org).*

6. Differential diagnostics

Differential diagnosis includes Dengue fever, Chikungunya virus, West Nile virus, Yellow fever, Malaria infection, Leptospirosis, Rubella, infectious Erythema (parvovirus B19 infection), Rocky Mountain spotted fever, Group A streptococcal infection, alphavirus infections, and coronavirus disease 2019 (COVID-19) [15–41]. Also, Mayaro, and the proposed ChikDenMaZika syndrome should be considered in the differential diagnostics [15–41].

7. Treatment of ZIKV disease

There is no specific treatment for ZIKV infection [15–43], and current treatment recommendations are based on limited evidence [15–44]. Thus, as with other mosquito-borne flaviviruses, treatment for ZIKV infection is symptomatic and supportive and includes [15–45]:

7.1 Symptomatic and supportive treatment

- Rest and adequate hydration.
- Use of analgesics or antipyretics: Acetaminophen 325–1000 mg orally every 4 to 6 hours when necessary (maximum 4000 mg/day). Aspirin and other non-steroidal anti-inflammatory drugs (NSAIDs) should be avoided until dengue virus infection has been ruled out, to reduce the risk of bleeding.
- Calamine lotion can be used for the maculopapular rash.

*The management of pregnant women, congenital Zika syndrome, and Guillain-Barré syndrome is described in detail elsewhere [15–41].

Although a large number of existing drugs and novel chemical compounds have been postulated as possible interventions against ZIKV [15–46] and some have shown activity against ZIKV in animal and experimental models [15–48], none have yet demonstrated safety and efficacy in clinical trials [15-49]. A safety and tolerability trial for the monoclonal antibody against ZIKV called Tyzivumab (NCT03443830), and another for a polyclonal antibody against ZIKV (NCT03624946) have completed their recruitment phase and are currently in progress. At the moment, there are no treatments approved by government agencies for ZIKV, and there is no information to suggest that there are treatments in advanced stages of development [20–40].

8. Advances in vaccination

Significant efforts have been made to develop safe and effective vaccines against ZIKV. International scientific cooperation has resulted in multiple candidate vaccines that are now in various stages of clinical and preclinical development [22–42]. Several vaccines are being developed, including purified inactivated viral particles (PIV), purified virus-like particles (VLPs) and viral subunit proteins, live attenuated vaccines, chimeric vaccines, and viral and non-viral vectors that encode ZIKV structural proteins [20–43]. The most advanced candidate corresponds to a DNA vaccine (VRC5283) developed by the National Institute of Allergy and Infectious Diseases (NIAID) that is being evaluated in phase 2 clinical study (NCT03110770) that seeks to evaluate the safety and tolerability of the vaccine. (Phase A) and the safety and efficacy compared to placebo (Phase B); that is, the safety, immunogenicity, optimal dose of administration are evaluated, and an attempt will be made to determine the ability of the vaccine to prevent the disease caused by ZIKV infection effectively. At the time of this writing, the results published on www.clinical.trials.gov had not completed the quality control review process. However, its results have been promising [20–44]. However, significant challenges remain in the development of vaccines for ZIKV. Difficulties include the heterogeneity of the incidence of ZIKV infection, difficulties in financing, regulation and authorisation of vaccines, which in turn has limited the conduct of phase 2 and 3 clinical trials and prompted international organisations to consider approaches alternative, as models of infection by controlled human exposure [25–46]. Vaccine development for ZIKV is underway.

9. Conclusions

The impact and burden of Zika in the Americas region have multiple implications. Clinical and epidemiological research has been vital in the understanding and developing of knowledge for the management and prevention of this emerging arboviral disease [30–48]. Still, many challenges exist, including the developing of an effective vaccine, still under developing.

Author details

Carlos Andrés Rosero-Oviedo[1], D. Katterine Bonilla-Aldana[2,3], Jaime A. Cardona-Ospina[1,2,4], Wilmer E. Villamil-Gómez[5,6] and Alfonso J. Rodriguez-Morales[1,2,3,4,5*]

1 Grupo de Investigación Biomedicina, Faculty of Medicine, Fundación Universitaria Autónoma de las Américas, Pereira, Risaralda, Colombia

2 Public Health and Infection Research Group, Faculty of Health Sciences, Universidad Tecnológica de Pereira, Pereira, Colombia

3 Semillero de Investigación en Zoonosis, Grupo BIOECOS, Fundación Universitaria Autónoma de las Américas, Pereira, Colombia

4 Emerging Infectious Diseases and Tropical Medicine Research Group, Instituto para la Investigación en Ciencias Biomédicas-Sci-Help, Pereira, Colombia

5 Infectious Diseases and Infection Control Research Group, Hospital Universitario de Sincelejo, Sincelejo, Sucre, Colombia

6 Programa del Doctorado de Medicina Tropical, SUE Caribe, Universidad del Atlántico, Barranquilla, Colombia

*Address all correspondence to: ajrodriguezmmd@gmail.com

References

[1] DICK, G. W. (1953). Epidemiological notes on some viruses isolated in Uganda; Yellow fever, Rift Valley fever, Bwamba fever, West Nile, Mengo, Semliki forest, Bunyamwera, Ntaya, Uganda S and Zika viruses. Transactions of the Royal Society of Tropical Medicine and Hygiene, Jan;47(1), 13-48. https://doi.org/10.1016/0035-9203(53)90021-2

[2] DICK, G. W., KITCHEN, S. F., & HADDOW, A. J. (1952). Zika virus. I. Isolations and serological specificity. Transactions of the Royal Society of Tropical Medicine and Hygiene, Sep;46(5), 509-20. https://doi.org/10.1016/0035-9203(52)90042-4

[3] DICK, G. W. (1952). Zika virus. II. Pathogenicity and physical properties. Transactions of the Royal Society of Tropical Medicine and Hygiene, Sep;46(5), 521-34. https://doi.org/10.1016/0035-9203(52)90043-6

[4] Campos, G. S., Bandeira, A. C., & Sardi, S. I. (2015). Zika Virus Outbreak, Bahia, Brazil. Emerging Infectious Diseases, Oct;21(10), 1885-1886. https://doi.org/10.3201/eid2110.150847

[5] Schuler-Faccini, L., Ribeiro, E. M., Feitosa, I. M., Horovitz, D. D., Cavalcanti, D. P., Pessoa, A., Doriqui, M. J., Neri, J. I., Neto, J. M., Wanderley, H. Y., Cernach, M., El-Husny, A. S., Pone, M. V., Serao, C. L., Sanseverino, M. T., & Brazilian Medical Genetics Society–Zika Embryopathy Task Force (2016). Possible Association Between Zika Virus Infection and Microcephaly - Brazil, 2015. MMWR. Morbidity and mortality weekly report, 65(3), 59-62. https://doi.org/10.15585/mmwr.mm6503e2

[6] Camacho, E., Paternina-Gomez, M., Blanco, P. J., Osorio, J. E., & Aliota, M. T. (2016). Detection of Autochthonous Zika Virus Transmission in Sincelejo, Colombia. Emerging infectious diseases, 22(5), 927-929. https://doi.org/10.3201/eid2205.160023

[7] Sarmiento-Ospina, A., Vásquez-Serna, H., Jimenez-Canizales, C. E., Villamil-Gómez, W. E., & Rodriguez-Morales, A. J. (2016). Zika virus associated deaths in Colombia. The Lancet. Infectious diseases, 16(5), 523-524. https://doi.org/10.1016/S1473-3099(16)30006-8

[8] WHO statement on the first meeting of the International Health Regulations (2005) (IHR 2005) Emergency Committee on Zika virus and observed increase in neurological disorders and neonatal malformations. (2016). Retrieved November 23, 2020, from World Health Organization (WHO) website: https://www.who.int/news/item/01-02-2016-who-statement-on-the-first-meeting-of-the-international-health-regulations-(2005)-(ihr-2005)-emergency-committee-on-zika-virus-and-observed-increase-in-neurological-disorders-and-neonatal-malformations

[9] Zika situation report. (2016). Retrieveded November 23, 2020, from World Health Organization (WHO) website: https://www.who.int/emergencies/zika-virus/situation-report/31-march-2016/en/

[10] Zika epidemiology update. (2019). Retrieveded November 23, 2020, from World Health Organization (WHO) website: https://www.who.int/emergencies/diseases/zika/epidemiology-update/en/

[11] Simmonds, P., Becher, P., Bukh, J., Gould, E. A., Meyers, G., Monath, T., Muerhoff, S., Pletnev, A., Rico-Hesse, R., Smith, D. B., Stapleton, J. T., & Ictv Report Consortium (2017). ICTV Virus Taxonomy Profile: Flaviviridae. The Journal of general virology, 98(1), 2-3. https://doi.org/10.1099/jgv.0.000672

[12] Kuno, G., Chang, G. J., Tsuchiya, K. R., Karabatsos, N., & Cropp, C. B. (1998). Phylogeny of the genus Flavivirus. Journal of virology, 72(1), 73-83. https://doi.org/10.1128/JVI.72.1.73-83.1998

[13] Gutiérrez-Bugallo, G., Piedra, L. A., Rodriguez, M., Bisset, J. A., Lourenço-de-Oliveira, R., Weaver, S. C., Vasilakis, N., & Vega-Rúa, A. (2019). Vector-borne transmission and evolution of Zika virus. Nature ecology & evolution, 3(4), 561-569. https://doi.org/10.1038/s41559-019-0836-z

[14] Gregory, C. J., Oduyebo, T., Brault, A. C., Brooks, J. T., Chung, K. W., Hills, S., Kuehnert, M. J., Mead, P., Meaney-Delman, D., Rabe, I., Staples, E., & Petersen, L. R. (2017). Modes of Transmission of Zika Virus. The Journal of infectious diseases, 216(suppl_10), S875–S883. https://doi.org/10.1093/infdis/jix396

[15] Grischott, F., Puhan, M., Hatz, C., & Schlagenhauf, P. (2016). Non-vector-borne transmission of Zika virus: A systematic review. Travel medicine and infectious disease, 14(4), 313-330.

[16] BEARCROFT W. G. (1956). Zika virus infection experimentally induced in a human volunteer. Transactions of the Royal Society of Tropical Medicine and Hygiene, 50(5), 442-448.

[17] Baud, D., Gubler, D. J., Schaub, B., Lanteri, M. C., & Musso, D. (2017). An update on Zika virus infection. Lancet (London, England), 390(10107), 2099-2109. https://doi.org/10.1016/S0140-6736(17)31450-2

[18] Duffy, M. R., Chen, T. H., Hancock, W. T., Powers, A. M., Kool, J. L., Lanciotti, R. S., Pretrick, M., Marfel, M., Holzbauer, S., Dubray, C., Guillaumot, L., Griggs, A., Bel, M., Lambert, A. J., Laven, J., Kosoy, O., Panella, A., Biggerstaff, B. J., Fischer, M., & Hayes, E. B. (2009). Zika virus outbreak on Yap Island, Federated States of Micronesia. The New England journal of medicine, 360(24), 2536-2543. https://doi.org/10.1056/NEJMoa0805715

[19] Aubry, M., Teissier, A., Huart, M., Merceron, S., Vanhomwegen, J., Roche, C., Vial, A. L., Teururai, S., Sicard, S., Paulous, S., Desprès, P., Manuguerra, J. C., Mallet, H. P., Musso, D., Deparis, X., & Cao-Lormeau, V. M. (2017). Zika Virus Seroprevalence, French Polynesia, 2014-2015. Emerging infectious diseases, 23(4), 669-672. https://doi.org/10.3201/eid2304.161549

[20] Krow-Lucal, E. R., Biggerstaff, B. J., & Staples, J. E. (2017). Estimated Incubation Period for Zika Virus Disease. Emerging infectious diseases, 23(5), 841-845. https://doi.org/10.3201/eid2305.161715

[21] Musso, D., & Gubler, D. J. (2016). Zika Virus. Clinical microbiology reviews, 29(3), 487-524.

[22] Plourde, A. R., & Bloch, E. M. (2016). A Literature Review of Zika Virus. Emerging infectious diseases, 22(7), 1185-1192. https://doi.org/10.3201/eid2207.151990

[23] Cardona-Ospina, J. A., Henao-SanMartin, V., Acevedo-Mendoza, W. F., Nasner-Posso, K. M., Martínez-Pulgarín, D. F., Restrepo-López, A., Valencia-Gallego, V., Collins, M. H., & Rodriguez-Morales, A. J. (2019). Fatal Zika virus infection in the Americas: A systematic review. International journal of infectious diseases, 88, 49-59. https://doi.org/10.1016/j.ijid.2019.08.033

[24] Ximenes, R., Ramsay, L. C., Miranda, R. N., Morris, S. K., Murphy, K., Sander, B., & RADAM-LAC Research Team (2019). Health outcomes associated with Zika virus infection in humans: a systematic review of systematic reviews. BMJ open, 9(11), e032275. https://doi.org/10.1136/bmjopen-2019-032275

[25] Identification and management of Guillain-Barré syndrome in the context of Zika virus Interim guidance. (2016). Retrieved November 23, 2020, from World Health Organization (WHO) website: https://www.who.int/csr/resources/publications/zika/guillain-barre-syndrome/en/

[26] Lanciotti, R. S., Kosoy, O. L., Laven, J. J., Velez, J. O., Lambert, A. J., Johnson, A. J., Stanfield, S. M., & Duffy, M. R. (2008). Genetic and serologic properties of Zika virus associated with an epidemic, Yap State, Micronesia, 2007. Emerging infectious diseases, 14(8), 1232-1239.

[27] Zika virus disease Interim case definition. (2016). Retrieved November 23, 2020, from World Health Organization (WHO) website: https://www.who.int/csr/disease/zika/case-definition/en/

[28] Furtado, G., & Scavuzzi, A. (2020). Zika virus infection. Retrieved November 23, 2020, from BMJ Best Practice website: https://bestpractice.bmj.com/topics/en-us/1302

[29] Clinical Evaluation & Disease. (2019). Retrieved November 23, 2020, from Centers for Disease Control and Prevention (CDC) website: https://www.cdc.gov/zika/hc-providers/preparing-for-zika/clinicalevaluationdisease.html

[30] Zika virus. (2018). Retrieved November 23, 2020, from World Health Organization (WHO) website: https://www.who.int/news-room/fact-sheets/detail/zika-virus

[31] Epidemiological Update, Zika virus infection. (2015). Recuperado 23 de noviembre de 2020, de Pan American Health Organization (PAHO) website: https://iris.paho.org/handle/10665.2/50667

[32] LaBeaud, A. D. (2020). Zika virus infection: An overview. Retrieved November 23, 2020, from UpToDate website: https://www.uptodate.com/contents/zika-virus-infection-an-overview

[33] Barrows, N. J., Campos, R. K., Powell, S. T., Prasanth, K. R., Schott-Lerner, G., Soto-Acosta, R., Galarza-Muñoz, G., McGrath, E. L., Urrabaz-Garza, R., Gao, J., Wu, P., Menon, R., Saade, G., Fernandez-Salas, I., Rossi, S. L., Vasilakis, N., Routh, A., Bradrick, S. S., & Garcia-Blanco, M. A. (2016). A Screen of FDA-Approved Drugs for Inhibitors of Zika Virus Infection. Cell host & microbe, 20(2), 259-270.

[34] Bernatchez, J. A., Tran, L. T., Li, J., Luan, Y., Siqueira-Neto, J. L., & Li, R. (2020). Drugs for the Treatment of Zika Virus Infection. Journal of medicinal chemistry, 63(2), 470-489.

[35] Gorshkov, K., Shiryaev, S. A., Fertel, S., Lin, Y. W., Huang, C. T., Pinto, A., Farhy, C., Strongin, A. Y., Zheng, W., & Terskikh, A. V. (2019). Zika Virus: Origins, Pathological Action, and Treatment Strategies. Frontiers in microbiology, 9, 3252.

[36] G Viveiros Rosa, S., Fierro, I. M., & C Santos, W. (2020). Repositioning and investigational drugs for Zika virus infection treatment: a patent review. Expert opinion on therapeutic patents, 30(11), 847-862. https://doi.org/10.1080/13543776.2020.1811854

[37] Zika Virus Response Updates from FDA. (2020). Retrieved November 23, 2020, from United States Food and Drug Administration (FDA) website: https://www.fda.gov/emergency-preparedness-and-response/mcm-issues/zika-virus-response-updates-fda

[38] Abbink, P., Stephenson, K. E., & Barouch, D. H. (2018). Zika virus vaccines. Nature reviews. Microbiology, 16(10), 594-600.

[39] Pattnaik, A., Sahoo, B. R., & Pattnaik, A. K. (2020). Current Status of Zika Virus Vaccines: Successes and Challenges. Vaccines, 8(2), 266.

[40] Poland, G. A., Kennedy, R. B., Ovsyannikova, I. G., Palacios, R., Ho, P. L., & Kalil, J. (2018). Development of vaccines against Zika virus. The Lancet. Infectious diseases, 18(7), e211–e219.

[41] Gaudinski, M. R., Houser, K. V., Morabito, K. M., Hu, Z., Yamshchikov, G., Rothwell, R. S., Berkowitz, N., Mendoza, F., Saunders, J. G., Novik, L., Hendel, C. S., Holman, L. A., Gordon, I. J., Cox, J. H., Edupuganti, S., McArthur, M. A., Rouphael, N. G., Lyke, K. E., Cummings, G. E., Sitar, S., ... VRC 320 study teams (2018). Safety, tolerability, and immunogenicity of two Zika virus DNA vaccine candidates in healthy adults: randomised, open-label, phase 1 clinical trials. Lancet (London, England), 391(10120), 552-562.

[42] Wilder-Smith, A., Vannice, K., Durbin, A., Hombach, J., Thomas, S. J., Thevarjan, I., & Simmons, C. P. (2018). Zika vaccines and therapeutics: landscape analysis and challenges ahead. BMC medicine, 16(1), 84.

[43] Sharp TM, Fischer M, Muñoz-Jordán JL, Paz-Bailey G, Staples JE, Gregory CJ, Waterman SH. Dengue and Zika Virus Diagnostic Testing for Patients with a Clinically Compatible Illness and Risk for Infection with Both Viruses. MMWR Recomm Rep. 2019 Jun 14;68(1):1-10. doi: 10.15585/mmwr.rr6801a1.

[44] Rodriguez-Morales AJ, Villamil-Gómez WE, Franco-Paredes C. The arboviral burden of disease caused by co-circulation and co-infection of dengue, chikungunya and Zika in the Americas. Travel Med Infect Dis. 2016 May-Jun;14(3):177-179.

[45] Villamil-Gómez WE, Mendoza-Guete A, Villalobos E, González-Arismendy E, Uribe-García AM, Castellanos JE, Rodríguez-Morales AJ. Diagnosis, management and follow-up of pregnant women with Zika virus infection: A preliminary report of the ZIKERNCOL cohort study on Sincelejo, Colombia. Travel Med Infect Dis. 2016 Mar-Apr;14(2):155-158.

[46] Arzuza-Ortega L, Polo A, Pérez-Tatis G, López-García H, Parra E, Pardo-Herrera LC, Rico-Turca AM, Villamil-Gómez W, Rodríguez-Morales AJ. Fatal Sickle Cell Disease and Zika Virus Infection in Girl from Colombia.Emerg Infect Dis 2016 May; 22(5):925-927.

[47] Villamil-Gomez WE, Sánchez-Herrera ÁR, Hernandez H, Hernández-Iriarte J, Díaz-Ricardo K, Castellanos J, de Jesús Villamil-Macareno W, Rodriguez-Morales AJ. Guillain-Barré syndrome during the Zika virus outbreak in Sucre, Colombia, 2016. Travel Med Infect Dis. 2017;16:62-63.

[48] Paniz-Mondolfi AE, Rodriguez-Morales AJ, Blohm G, Marquez M, Villamil-Gomez WE. ChikDenMaZika Syndrome: the challenge of diagnosing arboviral infections in the midst of concurrent epidemics. Ann Clin Microbiol Antimicrob. 2016 Jul 22; 15:42.

[49] Oduyebo T, Polen KD, Walke HT, Reagan-Steiner S, Lathrop E, Rabe IB, Kuhnert-Tallman WL, Martin SW, Walker AT, Gregory CJ, Ades EW, Carroll DS, Rivera M, Perez-Padilla J, Gould C, Nemhauser JB, Ben Beard C, Harcourt JL, Viens L, Johansson M, Ellington SR, Petersen E, Smith LA, Reichard J, Munoz-Jordan J, Beach MJ, Rose DA, Barzilay E, Noonan-Smith M, Jamieson DJ, Zaki SR, Petersen LR, Honein MA, Meaney-Delman D. Update: Interim Guidance for Health Care Providers Caring for Pregnant Women with Possible Zika Virus Exposure - United States (Including U.S. Territories), July 2017. MMWR Morb Mortal Wkly Rep. 2017 Jul 28;66(29):781-793. doi: 10.15585/mmwr.mm6629e1.

Chapter 2

Risk Management of Zika in Context of Medical Provision and in Favor of Disaster Medicine: New Opportunities for Risk Reduction (The Conceptual Idea)

Diana Dimitrova

Abstract

There is a need for timely medical care to the population for the risk management of Zika nowadays. Although scientists determine the widespread nature of the worldwide outbreak of Zika virus infection, it seems clear that there is a real need for outside help to deal with this disease. The Zika disease affects predominantly negatively the fetus in pregnant women, but cases of severe clinical manifestations are also reported among adults. Irrespective of age, it is known to affect the nervous system in humans. The vector causes epidemiological data to expand its area of expertise. In this light of expression, specialists define and attribute to this disease the type and significance of a worldwide disaster management. This requires an in-depth study and analysis of risk factors and their management as a fundamental approach for their prevention and for the benefit of disaster medicine. Reducing the risk with existing traditional tools and methods is not enough to meet the growing needs of people and territories at risk of Zika infection. New strategy approaches and technologies are being sought, and new risk reduction (RR) options are being interpreted. A framework for an innovative conceptual idea based on nano-biotechnology for risk reduction and prevention for Zika virus infection is presented.

Keywords: Zika, risk management, risk reduction, prevention measures (with SWOT analysis), medical provision of the population, disaster medicine, innovative conceptual idea, nano-biotechnology

1. Introduction

The World Health Organization (WHO) has declared the Zika infection an international threat to public health since the beginning of February 2016 [1–3]. The definition, classification, and analysis of the risk factors of the evolution and spread of Zika virus infection require the proper application in time and space of known preventive measures, as well as measures for the protection and medical provision of the population. The real challenge nowadays is to meet the growing demands of society, expanding the opportunities for highly effective risk reduction (RR) and incorporating new technological and strategic solutions to achieve rapid results.

IntechOpen

2. Data and analyses of Zika in favor of risk reduction conception

2.1 Epidemiology and the spread of Zika virus: facts and analyses

It is a well-known fact that the Zika virus belongs to the *Flaviviridae* family of the genus *Flavivirus* [1]. The data indicate that the Zika virus was isolated in 1947 from Macaque monkeys in Uganda in the Uganda Forest to which it is named [1, 4, 5]. Retrospective analysis shows that the Zika virus was first studied by scientists at the Yellow Fever Institute (founded in 1936). Later, in 1948, the Zika virus was isolated for the second time in the tiger mosquito. Scientists have discovered the first manifestations of the infection by observing the effects of the virus on the Macaque monkey. Subsequently, the virus was isolated from the blood serum [4, 5]. During the next few years, the Zika virus underwent serious studies and in 1952 received its name in the virological nomenclature. In the International Classification of Diseases, ICD-10 is described under the code name A92.8 [6]. In humans, the virus is known to be the cause of the disease known as Zika fever or Zika disease, spreading since 1950 from *Africa* to *Asia* [7, 8].

Firstly, the data indicate that in 2014, the virus was *transmitted* across the *Pacific* to *French Polynesia*, reaching the shores of Easter Island. Secondly, the surveillance of Zika virus infection since the beginning of 2016 indicates an intensive *epidemic boom* with increasing prevalence of the disease in El Salvador, Venezuela, Colombia, Brazil, Suriname, French Guiana, Honduras, Mexico, Panama, and Martinique. Thirdly, in 2015 there were reported cases in Central America, the Caribbean, and South America, where Zika caused the development of a *pandemic*. It is also known that *sporadic* cases in Guatemala, Paraguay, Puerto Rico, Barbados, St. Martin, and Haiti are reported. According to the World Health Organization, Zika is spreading explosively and could affect 3–4 million people in the Americas. Furthermore, it is believed that the Zika virus was unknown to the US region prior to 2015. Finally, a retrospective analysis of the data indicates that nowadays Zika fever is a serious socially significant disease in the *US region* for which the resources available for its prevention, treatment, and control are scarce [1, 4, 5, 9, 10].

In 2013, there have been cases reported of the disease in *Europe* as well. From South America, tourists carry the virus to Europe. Ten Zika fever (ZVD) cases have been reported in Germany since 2013. There are four in Italy, three in the UK, and seven in Spain in the Zika virus case, as well as one case each in Sweden and Denmark. It is possible that the number of Europeans infected with Zika is much larger without themselves knowing it. According to the American Center for Disease Control and Prevention (CDCP), only one in five people infected with the virus develops the disease. The southern part of the European continent is generally of moderate risk for ZVD. The risk of Zika spreading in Europe in late spring and summer is described as "small to moderate," according to the WHO. The Zika virus is "highly likely" to spread to three European regions where there are tiger mosquitoes that carry it. These are the Portuguese island of Madeira in the Atlantic Ocean and the Russian and Georgian Black Sea coasts. For the other 18 predominantly Mediterranean countries, including Spain, France, Italy, Croatia, Greece, and Turkey, the risk is mostly considered moderate. According to the data provided by the WHO on the spread of Zika, the territory of Bulgaria is identified to be a moderate-risk country for this disease. Analysis of data from the World Meteorological Organization (WMO), the National Institute of Meteorology and Hydrology (NIMH) in Bulgaria, and the Institute for Atmospheric, Climate and Water Research (IACWR) at BAS (functioning from January 1, 2019) in Bulgaria about humidity, high summer temperatures, and the average altitude of the entire terrain of Southern Europe shows the increasing number of mosquitoes spreading the Zika virus [1, 9, 11–14].

2.2 Vectors facts and analyses of spreading ZVD

The infection is known to be transmitted to humans through the bite of infected mosquitoes of the *Aedes* family, most commonly the species *Aedes aegypti* and *Aedes albopictus* or the "Asian tiger mosquito." It seems that these two species are widespread in the tropical regions of Asia, Africa, and America. In fact, the tiger mosquitoes are native to Southeast Asia. The Zika virus was also isolated from *A. africanus*, *A. apicoargenteus*, *A. furcifer*, *A. hensilli*, *A. luteocephalus*, and *A. vittatus*. Generally, tiger mosquitoes can transmit dangerous viral and parasitic diseases to humans and pets, including *Zika*, yellow fever, St. Louis encephalitis, West Nile encephalitis, chikungunya, dengue, heartworm (in dogs and cats), and others [1, 3–5, 11, 15–19].

In *the USA*, it was proven in 1985 in Texas and Maine; in Hawaii in 1986; in Brazil, Argentina, and Mexico in 1988; in the Dominican Republic in 1993; in Paraguay in 1999; in Panama in 2002; and in Uruguay and Nicaragua 2003 [1–5, 17, 18].

It penetrated South *Africa* in 1990, Nigeria in 1991, Cameroon in 1999, and Gabon in 2006 [1, 4, 5, 10, 19] and *in the Middle East*—Lebanon and Israel in 2003 and Syria in 2005 [4, 5, 19].

The Asian mosquito originates from tropical and subtropical regions of Southeast *Asia* [1, 9, 10, 19]. In the last few decades, it has spread to many other regions of the world mainly through means of transport and intensive commodity trade. It was brought to *Europe* in 1979 in Albania in goods from China and has begun to spread massively along *the Mediterranean coast* since 1990. In 1990–1991 it was established in Italy, transported in old tires from the USA, and spread throughout the country, including the islands of Sicily and Sardinia. In 1999 it reached southern France and the island of Corsica. Other countries affected were Belgium in 2000–2001; Montenegro in 2003; Switzerland and Greece in 2004; Spain and Croatia in 2005; the Netherlands, Bosnia and Herzegovina, and Slovenia in 2006; Germany in 2007; Greece (in areas close to or adjacent to Bulgaria) in 2008; and Malta in 2010 [1, 4, 5, 9–11, 19].

In 2011, the presence of a tiger mosquito in *Bulgaria*, in Sozopol (Burgas region), was first established. In 2014 it was detected in Burgas and Plovdiv. In January 2016, there were also data on the spread of the disease vector in Bulgaria in the districts of Blagoevgrad, Pazardzhik, Varna, Vratsa, Montana, Plovdiv, and Stara Zagora. The risk of expansion of the territory in the Danube Plain and in the Upper Thracian Plain and the valleys of the Struma and Mesta rivers is real and is defined as high for the country during the warm months of the year [11, 19, 20].

According to the WHO, *the Black Sea coast* is among the most endangered areas in Europe in the spread of Asian tiger mosquito. The potential risk is identified in all territories [1, 11, 19, 20].

It is also known that the spread of mosquitoes, which causes the transmission of the Zika virus, develops in places with an altitude of up to 200 m. An interesting fact is that mosquitoes attack during the day, prefer humans over other warm-blooded animals, and hide and breed close to human homes [19, 20].

Research shows that mosquitoes are the only carriers of the pathogen, and the Zika virus infection can mainly spread to humans and monkeys. There is a serious risk of spreading the infection only if the viral infection spreads through humans and mosquitoes from areas of normal habitat to the European continent. This spread can be done by sick people arriving from Africa and America or by the direct infestation of mosquitoes from infected areas [1, 11, 19, 20].

2.3 The Zika fever facts and analyses

Studies show that the incubation period of the Zika virus is about 10 days; mostly it is known that people get infected first and foremost by tiger mosquito *bites* (Zika virus carrier). Some data indicated that ZVD can spread to other people through *sexual contact* and is directly infused and inoculated in the placenta [1, 2, 19].

The first case of a possible Zika virus *transfusion* in 2014 at the Hematology Center at Campinas University in São Paulo has also been reported [2, 7, 19].

The virus has been shown to damage the human nervous system and infect, damage, and kill the cells of the developing human brain even more prenatally, disrupting the localization of a pTBK1-protein, the protein that helps in cell division of the growing brain. The scientific community also discusses the link between Zika and microcephaly or congenital anomalies in newborns whose mothers became ill with the Zika virus during pregnancy. After 2014, the disease is associated with Guillain-Barré syndrome, which has been reported in some of the patients with ZVD [15–20].

2.4 Classification and analysis of Zika-related risk factors (author analysis)

The epidemiological data and the facts and analyses for the development and spread of the Zika vector and Zika virus are a good basis for elucidating Zika-related risk factors. Knowledge of risk factors, in turn, enables us to group them according to their type and nature and to give an idea of their classification. This is in favor of building a concise idea of a concept for the possibilities of the reduction and prevention of ZVDs at different levels and stages according to the specific needs and according to the stage of development of the disease from the moment of entry to the person in the distribution zone of Zika vector to the incidence of Zika virus in the human body.

2.4.1 From current conclusions to the conceptual models of ZVD (author analysis)

Nowadays the knowledge that we have about Zika virus infection provides us with some generalizing current conclusions that promise a better understanding of some conceptual models of Zika virus infection (**Figure 1**).

1. Zika fever is a vector-borne disease [1–22].

2. The Zika virus infection vector is also a vector of many other pathogenic viruses and parasites.

3. Practically, the vector spreads under high humidity and moderately high temperature at low altitude.

4. The vector is adaptive and easily enters new habitats through the transport of goods and passengers, mainly by means of water, rapidly increasing its population in warm and humid weather.

5. Climate change provides new threats to humans and new territories for the spread of the vector.

6. The virus spreads in parallel with the area of development and propagation of its vector but does not necessarily exist in all cases of typical habitat of its vector.

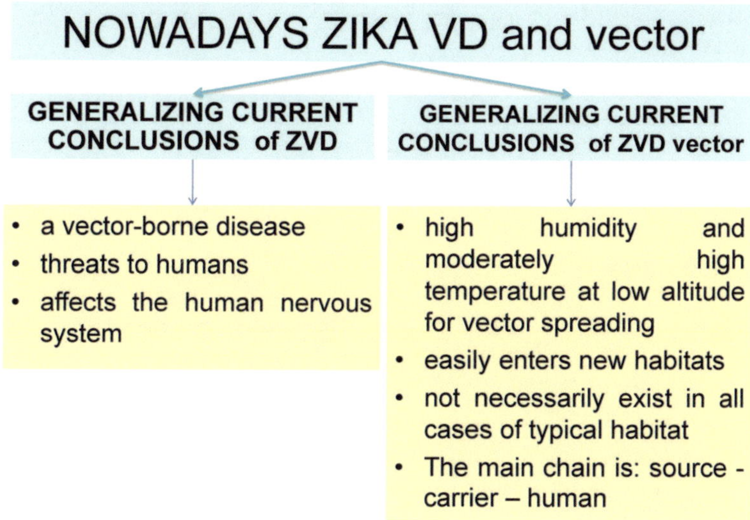

Figure 1.
Zika VD and Zika vector.

7. A prerequisite for the development of Zika fever besides the vector is the presence of a source in a susceptible population by a few chains.

8. The chain of infection with ZVDs can be represented in a few types. The main chain is source-carrier-human. Another chain is also possible: man-man in a vertical and horizontal direction. This is explained by the transplacental transfer (intrauterine infection) of the virus from the pregnant woman to the embryo and fetus, as well as by the transfusion of biological fluids physiologically or mechanically.

9. The virus affects the human nervous system, but not necessarily every person infected with Zika virus infection.

10. Probably the human immune system does not have a good enough response in time and space to stop the damage to the nervous system in every case of infection.

During the study of Zika virus infection, the following several questions arose (**Figure 2**):

1. Is global climate change likely to increase the risk of people with Zika virus infection, and is it possible to reduce this threat?

2. Is it possible to reduce the risk of vector spread of Zika virus infection, and can the population of the vector be reduced by a competitive species or other natural species?

3. Is it possible a mosquito vector to lose its role as a vector?

4. Can the vector be tilted in such a way that it does not affect the person with the bites?

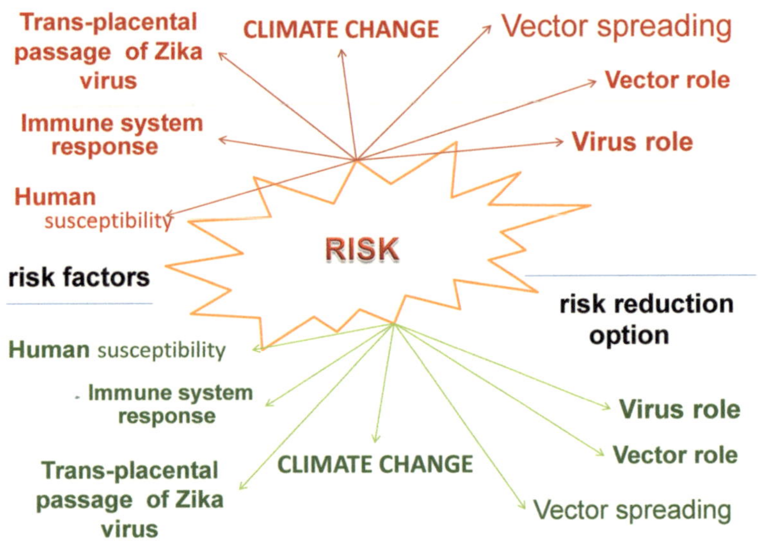

Figure 2.
New risk factors and risk reduction option.

5. Is it possible, if a mosquito bite (as a vector) humans, to stop the entry of Zika virus into the human body?

6. Is it possible to stop the Zika virus that has entered the human body during the bite of the vector?

7. Is it possible to reduce and/or completely stop human susceptibility to Zika virus?

8. Is it possible to understand the mechanism of the immune response in humans in which the Zika virus does not affect the nervous system, and are there other factors that support this course?

9. Is there a mechanism to support a person's immune response in such a way that no damage to the nervous system occurs?

10. Is it possible to prevent the transplacental passage of the Zika virus?

2.4.2 From groups of risk factors to the conceptual framework for modern technological approaches about ZVD (author analysis)

Some of the questions asked seem impossible and even naive in their search for possible solutions. However, the search for an answer, based on risk analysis, led slowly to the idea of a conceptual framework for modern technological approaches, in the hope of increasing the real chance of risk reduction in the process of risk management for the health provision of the population in favor of prevention and in the context of a disaster-prone process.

First of all, some groups of risk factors have emerged from a detailed examination of the available data on Zika virus infection [1–20].

According to the origin of their generation, there are two fundamental groups of risk factors, namely, natural and anthropogenic (**Figure 3**).

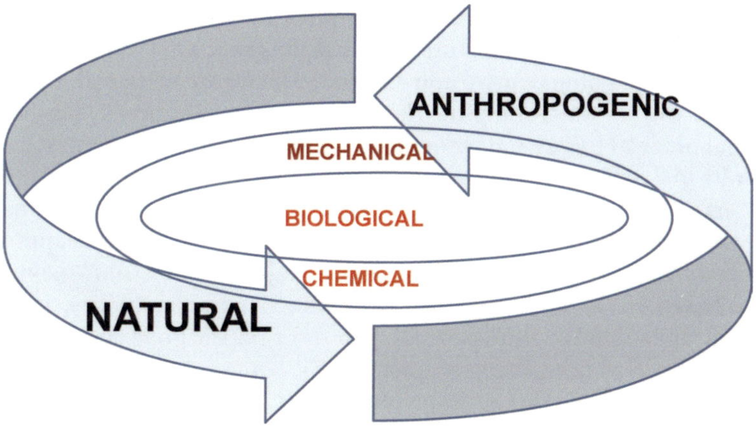

Figure 3.
Groups of risk factors.

Fundamental groups of risk factors can be divided into six main groups according to their type:

1. Risk factors arising from the environment (territorial risk factors, TRFs).

2. Risk factors resulting from the vector (VRFs).

3. Time and weather as risk factors (time risk factors).

4. Risk factors resulting from the population (receptivity, resistance, immune response).

5. Factors arising from human actions and/or inaction.

6. Factors related to knowledge and competence (scientific-cognitive) and the realization of ethical-legal and preventive-therapeutic ideas, methods, technologies, and concepts.

According to their mechanism, the risk factors can be selected as mechanical, physicochemical, and biochemical.

3. The Zika contemporary risk reduction conception

3.1 A brief look at preventive risk management measures (with SWOT analysis): from tradition to the future stage (author analysis)

Zika's strategic approaches about prevention are divided into three groups according to the moment of implementation of the specific tasks: before, during, and after the outbreak of the infection is occurred. In practice, these groups of methods are *strategic time-based approaches* to risk reduction. The timely application of this group of methods is also the responsibility for controlling the risk over time. On the other hand, the application of this approach leads to the reduction of disease territory, regression, and/or complete destruction of the risk areas (the occurrence of a hot and warm zone of infection within a particular territory) at a certain point in time. This is an important element of the health provision of the population (in a certain territory) over a period of time, not just the groups at risk, and is part of the national security. Ongoing control and extreme control are responsible for sporadic Zika infection and for controlling the risk of an epidemic outbreak. The inclusion of additional medical forces and resources when needed at a given time as a health policy results in a reduced response time to the massive nature of Zika disease in the short term. The specific aspects of this approach depend on the seasonality as well as the manifestations of the daily activity of the vector. The time approach is characterized by some cyclicality. Importantly, health-care decision-making considerations based on this approach require firmness, maneuverability, and agility. This strategic approach is a fundamental guarantor for the good control of the risk of Zika virus infection in a timely manner [1–27].

There are some known threats to invoking only these strategic time approaches. They are derived from the nature of the spread of the ZVD and namely through a vector. This requires that the health care of the population be stepped on the basis of *strategic territorial principle* [22] with emphasis on the environment and territory suitable for the development and dissemination of the vector. The control of the vector is possible and also depends on the close transinstitutional interaction, planning, and development of risk maps, as well as their strict updating and upgrading with new methods. Facilitated by appropriate local meteorological and global climate changes, the risk of a hot zone from a Zika virus is present and varies in extent and varies in space. The reduction and even destruction of the natural range of the vector undergo a health-sanitary control in collaboration with various professionals at every level of territorial division of the country—national, regional, and municipal levels. Cross-border cooperation is a fundamental step in the event of a high risk of spreading the disease outside the country. Migration and trans-oceanic transport of people and goods are factors facilitating the spread of the Zika disease. The globalization of the Zika disease proves the weaknesses of the territorial principle [1–20, 23–27].

Virus-based strategy, a strategic principle based on the viral genesis of the disease, the RNA genome of the causative agent, as well as its genetic variability, is being investigated. Insofar as there is predictability in specific parameters in the previous two principles, it is probabilistic in that. On the other hand, the creation of a specific vaccine and/or specific antiviral drug is a process of unknown duration, and time is proven to be an insufficient resource for the purpose of providing the population with medical care in the face of an epidemic. The laboratory demonstration of the virus both in vectors and in humans is an important step. However, the study and demonstration of Zika virus have its weaknesses, the main one being the recruitment of the necessary and sufficient scope of the study under the specific conditions for the construction of a strictly positive and strictly negative hypothesis for its presence. The process is time-consuming. The reliability of laboratory tests in terms of genomic variability of the virus requires both flexibility and a competitive environment for a prompt response by researchers and experts [1–20, 23–27].

Health education strategy for raising the health culture and awareness of both the population and health professionals is an approach complementary to the above, extending levels of responsibility to each individual except the medical services for the control of the spread of the Zika disease. Difficulties in making such information available to certain sections of the population in a country are defined as a weakness, as well as varying degrees of understanding of information submitted by each person at risk of being potentially affected. Access to health services is not equally available in all cases of the spread of the Zika disease. The levels of literacy and responsibility to one's own health are at different levels of manifestation [1–21, 23–27].

These four strategic approaches are classic approaches in nature. When used in combination, they produce significantly more reliable results (**Figure 4**).

Modern approaches, but with limited accessibility, are immunoprophylaxis approaches. They aim to enhance the immune response of the community, except for any member of the at-risk society. Approaches to *primary*, *secondary*, *or tertiary immunoprophylaxis* take wide limits. Immune protectors are gaining popularity. Immunomodulating herbal remedies complement and extend the boundaries of current immunoprophylactic approaches. Clinical homeopathy or allopathic homeopathy, phytotherapy, herbal medicine, etc. supplement the ability to stabilize and prepare the immune system to meet the Zika virus that is aggressive to the nervous system [1–20, 22–39].

Depending on their type [34], the methods can be grouped into both traditional (classical) and contemporary as well as progressively innovative. If traditional prophylaxis methods [28–31, 34–36] are environment-oriented [22, 37–39], vector-oriented [27, 36–38], or target-specific [21, 22, 35], or targeted at a susceptible population (potentially infected) [22, 38, 39], or a combination thereof, and contemporary to the human body's immune response or to the creation of high public immune status, then all these methods apply to society as a whole and have a group character.

3.2 Progressive-innovative approaches to reducing the risk of ZVD: technologies of the future stage (author's idea)

Innovative technologies excite science—quantum-based as well as nanotechnologies and related software models—supported by mathematical algorithms and block diagrams to model the framework of an innovative idea. In this regard, the Zika RNA virus, with its unknowns, predisposes us scientists to trying to solve the equation from another angle. It turns out that the actual scientific information on Zika is not satisfactory and requires the search for new approaches beyond the known ones in order to achieve more serious results and greater success in solving the equation with such unknowns. This is because if we apply the always known and recognized methods, we will always arrive at the same results. In this case, it means coming up with a specific vaccine and/or specific antiviral agent to deal with Zika disease. This is, of course, an excellent destination and also a well-known area for

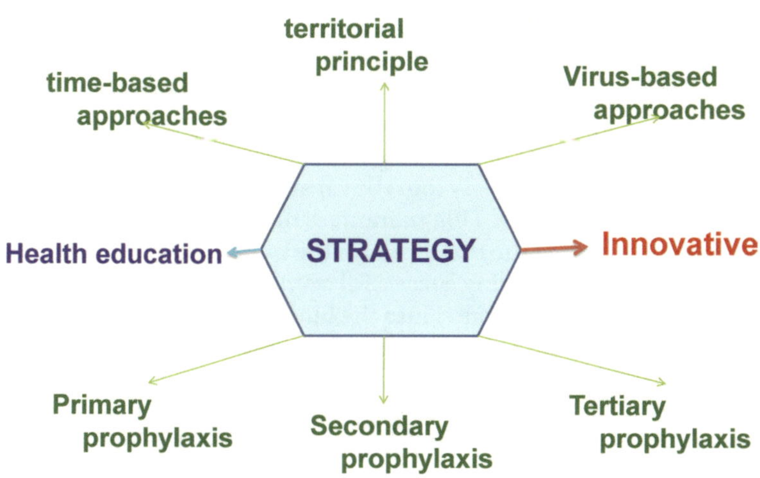

Figure 4.
Contemporary strategy of RR.

dealing with particularly dangerous infections. The high benefits of this approach have been proven, and this is because the world has dealt with diseases such as smallpox. The benefits are undeniable and highly appreciated. However, this is also not an obstacle to look for new approaches that could give another level of solutions. If we manage to integrate a new approach, although it may seem impossible and even absurd in its initial form as an idea, it may 1 day help to fundamentally tackle similar problems.

The thesis of the unrecognizability of Zika virus that has entered the human body appears as a counterbalance (counter thesis) to its recognition. In reality, heretofore, there is no known mechanism to protect the nervous system of the human body that is targeted by the Zika virus. Once penetrated into the body, the Zika virus takes several steps—to multiply, to cover the whole body, to cross the transplacental barrier, and to affect the nervous system and/or destroy it. Although initially recognized as an infectious agent by the immune system, it seems clear that the Zika virus is able to attack the nervous system both in the developing fetus during pregnancy and in some infected adults. The affinity of the virus to the nerve cell leads to its destruction and even to blocking its development in the embryo and fetus in pregnant women during the period of organogenesis. This makes the thesis of the unrecognizability of Zika virus relevant to the study.

The purpose and the tasks set have led us to the idea that biotechnological methods (in their varieties) can work for us in this direction. In reality, biotechnology gives us the opportunity to conduct research in the field of experience, as well as real-world attempts to solve the problem of early specific recognition of the Zika virus incorporated into the human body. The conceptual design covers several stages of its presentation, the most important of which is the targeted recognition of the Zika virus from the moment of the bite (from the mosquito carrier of the virus), through all steps of its incorporation, before it affects the nervous system and/or its development in the fetus.

The different levels of recognition create obstacles due to lack of information about the actual moment of the bite; ambiguity and unrecognition of nonspecific early symptoms; late identification of the disease; inaccessibility to medical services and early medical care; etc.

The invention and production of a nano-biotechnology carrier (as a conveyor) and its intravenous injection in order to determine whether a Zika virus has entered the human body as a key to dealing with the disease, before the virus strikes the nervous system, is a new type of idea. The capture of each virus in the shuttle (at the site of the bite, during their circulation in the body, or during its entry into the human cell) gives us a new opportunity to control the Zika virus. The implementation of this stage is supported by nano-biotechnology. The capture in the Zika shuttle of the virus in the human body requires sufficient durability to allow time for injection of substance "X" solely into the capsule of the virus from the carrier that has captured the Zika virus. This guarantees the destruction of the pathogenic virus only, without affecting the tissue cells in the human body. This is considered within the framework of achieving successful *secondary prophylaxis*, provided that the Zika virus is already incorporated into the human body or has serious clinical and/or laboratory indications of this in humans at risk. The therapeutic result will be available and delivered in a timely manner.

Moreover, the implementation of this approach can also be carried out in advance (as *primary prevention*) for any person who is at risk of being potentially bitten by a Zika virus vector carrier—researchers and scientists working in the field; field medical teams; emergency rescue teams; disaster, accident, and catastrophe field workers; etc. This will generate safety for the teams and enable rescue and rehabilitation activities on the worksite, as well as the successful completion of each mission in a Zika fever area, and will increase the chances of victims of emergency, disaster, accident, and catastrophe at risk of Zika fever. The time factor is in any case the basis for the successful completion of a given mission and/or field task at Zika's risk.

Preliminary studies of "X" substance on the effectiveness of the action to eradicate the pathogenic virus have been made. As far as one can tell, this substance can also be synthesized, except that it can be extracted from the natural sources of a precursor substance. It is assumed that there may be other variants of this substance and that there may be others that are effective, even with more potent action and with faster effect. However, in vivo and in vitro processes can sometimes show surprising results.

4. Conclusion

The idea presented as a theoretical formulation gives new horizons. It is clear that studies are still ongoing in the direction of effective control of the Zika virus. The aim is to demonstrate a mechanism or combination of methods and measures that can reduce the risk of the Zika virus as a possible result in the near future.

Conflict of interest

There are no "conflicts of interest."

Author details

Diana Dimitrova
Emergency CC, Department of EM and MCS, Stanke Dimitrov, Sofia, Bulgaria

*Address all correspondence to: d.dimitrova.phd.md@abv.bg

References

[1] WHO. Zika virus [Internet]. 2019. Available from: https://www.who.int/news-room/fact-sheets/detail/zika-virus

[2] WHO. Zika virus disease [Internet]. 2019. Available from: https://www.who.int/emergencies/diseases/zika/en/

[3] PAHO/WHO. Zika virus infection [Internet]. 2019. Available from: https://www.paho.org/hq/index.php%3Foption%3Dcom_topics%26view%3Darticle%2520%26id%3D427%26Itemid%3D41484%26lang%3Den

[4] WHO. Countries and territories with current or previous virus transmission [Internet]. 2019. Available from: https://www.who.int/emergencies/diseases/zika/countries-with-zika-and-vectors-table.pdf?ua=1

[5] Health Protection Surveillance Centre (HPSC). Zika virus infection—List of affected countries/areas [Internet]. 2019. Available from: https://www.hpsc.ie/a-z/vectorborne/zika/factsheet/listofaffectedcountries/

[6] WHO. International Classification of Diseases-ICD-10 [Internet]. 2019. Available from: https://www.who.int/classifications/icd/en/

[7] Zika virus. John Hopkins medicine [Internet]. 2019. Available from: https://www.hopkinsmedicine.org/zika-virus/what-is-zika-virus.html

[8] WHO. Zika virus disease. Interim case definitions [Internet]. 2016. Available from: https://apps.who.int/iris/bitstream/handle/10665/204381/WHO_ZIKV_SUR_16.1_eng.pdf;jsessionid=42E72E2D28DC1561ACA0E75F2E4CF639?sequence=1

[9] CDCP. Zika travel information [Internet]. 2019. Available from: https://wwwnc.cdc.gov/travel/page/zika-travel-information

[10] Center for Disease Control and Prevention (CDCP). Zika Virus, Statistics and Maps [Internet]. 2019. Available from: https://www.cdc.gov/zika/reporting/index.html

[11] European Center for Disease Prevention and Control. Environmental risk mapping: *Aedes albopictus* in Europe. Proof-of-concept study for the European environment and epidemiological network, Stockholm. Technical Report. 2013. DOI: 10.2900/78239. Available from: www.ecdc.europe.eu. ISBN: 978-92-9133-449-2

[12] World Meteorological Organization (WMO). Climate [Internet]. 2019. Available from: https://public.wmo.int/en/our-mandate/climate

[13] National Institute of Meteorology and Hydrology (NIMH) in Bulgaria [Internet]. Seasonal forecasts. 2019. Available from: http://www.weather.bg/0index.php?koiFail=seasonal&lng=1

[14] Institute for Atmospheric, Climate and Water Research (IACWR) at BAS in Bulgaria [Internet]. Country overview and assessment. 2019. Available from: https://ec.europa.eu/maritimeaffairs/sites/maritimeaffairs/files/docs/body/bulgaria_climate_change_en.pdf

[15] Leonhard SE, Lant S, Jacobs BC, et al. Zika virus infection in the returning traveller: What every neurologist should know. Practical Neurology. 2018;**18**:271-277. Available from: https://pn.bmj.com/content/practneurol/18/4/271.full.pdf

[16] Center for Disease Control and Prevention (CDCP). Zika Virus, Life Cycle: The Mosquito [Internet]. 2019. Available from: https://www.cdc.gov/zika/pdfs/MosquitoLifecycle.pdf

[17] Integrated Mosquito Management (IMM), Center for Disease Control and Prevention (CDCP). Zika Virus [Internet]. 2019. Available from: https://www.cdc.gov/zika/vector/integrated_mosquito_management.html

[18] Center for Disease Control and Prevention (CDCP). Zika Virus, Potential Range in US [Internet]. 2017. Available from: https://www.cdc.gov/zika/vector/range.html

[19] Zika. Bulgarian Red Cross [Internet]. 2019. Available from: http://www.redcross.bg/advice/zika.html

[20] Zika virus disease. NCIPD in Bulgaria, in Bulgarian [Internet]. 2019. Available from: https://www.ncipd.org/index.php?option=com_k2&view=item&id=255:zika-virusna-infektsia&lang=bg

[21] Dimitrova D. Medical provision of the population during Zika viral infection—Viral infections with mass medical losses. General Medicine. 2016;**18**(2):59-64

[22] World Health Organization. WHO guidelines for the prevention of sexual transmission of Zika virus: Executive summary. WHO/RHR/19.4; 2019

[23] Center for Disease Control and Prevention (CDCP). Zika Virus, Mosquito Control [Internet]. 2019. Available from: https://www.cdc.gov/zika/vector/index.html

[24] Center for Disease Control and Prevention (CDCP). Zika Virus, Controlling Mosquitoes at Home [Internet]. 2019. Available from: https://www.cdc.gov/zika/prevention/controlling-mosquitoes-at-home.html

[25] CDCP. Mosquito control activities by CDC to combat Zika virus transmission in the US. Draft programmatic environmental assessment [Internet]. 2017. Available from: https://www.cdc.gov/zika/pdfs/Draft-Environmental-Assessment-Mosquito-Control-for-publication.pdf

[26] Center for Disease Control and Prevention (CDCP). Zika Virus, Prevent Mosquito Bites [Internet]. 2019. Available from: https://www.cdc.gov/zika/prevention/prevent-mosquito-bites.html

[27] Guideline: Infant feeding in areas of Zika virus transmission. WHO Guidelines. ISBN: 978 92 4 154966 0

[28] Prevention of sexual transmission of Zika virus: Interim guidance update. WHO/ZIKV/MOC/16.1 Rev.3. Geneva: World Health Organization; 2016

[29] WHO Handbook for Guideline Development. 2nd ed. Geneva: World Health Organization; 2014

[30] WHO. Toolkit for the care and support of people affected by complications associated with Zika virus. ISBN: 978-92-4-151271-8

[31] MHNIM. Guidelines for Clinical Management, Laboratory Investigation and Surveillance of Patients with Zika Virus Infection. Ministry of Health, Nutrition & Indigenous Medicine, Sri Lanka; 2016

[32] Zika Virus Testing Guidelines for Healthcare Providers. Updated on 9/1/16

[33] Guidelines for classifying cases of Zika virus disease and related conditions. Global report. 2019

[34] WHO. Zika virus infection—Statutory notification. In: Public Health Management and Guidelines for Public Health Units. Global Overview. World Health Organization; 2019

[35] Epidemiological alert: Neurological syndrome, congenital malformations, and Zika virus infection. In:

Implications for Public Health in the Americas. Washington, DC: Pan American Health Organization, World Health Organization, Regional Office for the Americas; 2015

[36] Haddow AJ, Williams M, Woodall J, et al. Twelve isolations of Zika virus from *Aedes* (*Stegomyia*) *africanus* (*Theobald*) taken in and above a Uganda forest. Bulletin of the World Health Organization. 1964;**31**(1):57-69

[37] Thomas SM, Tjaden NB, van den Bos S, Beierkuhnlein C. Implementing cargo movement into climate based risk assessment of vector-borne diseases. International Journal of Environmental Research and Public Health AJPH. 2014;**11**(3):3360-3374

[38] MacDonald PDM, Wayne Holden E. Zika and public health: Understanding the epidemiology and information environment. Pediatrics. 2018;**141**(Suppl 2):S137-S145

[39] Howard Z. Zika virus. What New York State Clinicians Need to Know, NYS Commissioner of Health. 2016. Available from: https://www.health.ny.gov/diseases/zika_virus/docs/zika_webinar.pdf

Chapter 3

Animal Models of Zika Virus Sexual Transmission

Rafael K. Campos, Erin M. McDonald, Aaron C. Brault and Shannan L. Rossi

Abstract

ZIKV was first identified in the 1940s as a mosquito-borne virus; however, sexual transmission, which is uncommon for arboviruses, was demonstrated more than 60 years later. Tissue culture and animal models have allowed scientists to study how this transmission is possible. Immunocompromised mice infected with ZIKV had high viral loads in their testes, and infection of immunocompetent female mice was achieved following intravaginal inoculation or inoculation via mating with an infected male. These mouse studies lead researchers to investigate the individual components of the male reproductive system. In cell culture and mouse models, ZIKV can persist in Sertoli and germ cells of the testes and epithelial cells in the epididymis, which may lead to sexual transmission even after ZIKV has been cleared from other tissues. ZIKV has also been studied in nonhuman primates (NHPs), which appears to mimic the limited human epidemiological data, with low rates of symptomatic individuals and similar clinical signs. Although refinement is needed, these animal models have proven to be key in ZIKV research and continue to help uncovering the mechanisms of sexual transmission. This review will focus on the animal models used to elucidate the mechanisms of sexual transmission and persistence of flaviviruses.

Keywords: Zika virus, sexual transmission, animal models, human, primate, mouse, Sertoli cell, testes

1. Introduction

Zika virus (ZIKV) is a single-stranded, positive-sense virus of the genus *Flavivirus* of the family *Flaviviridae* that was discovered in the Ziika forest of Uganda in 1947 [1]. The virus was isolated during a surveillance campaign to attempt to identify yellow fever virus in the region. Sentinel rhesus macaques were placed in cages in the canopy layer of the trees and monitored daily for spikes in temperature. One of the rhesus macaques became febrile and was bled to isolate the causative agent of the fever. Serum from clarified blood caused illness when injected intra-cranially in white mice and the brain homogenates from these animals contained the first isolate of ZIKV, MR766. It is noteworthy that this strain, which is used in many contemporaneous studies, was passaged over 100 times in mice to increase its virulence in rodents. A second strain, ZIKV 758, was made from another rhesus macaque injected with homogenates of *Aedes africanus* mosquitoes collected in that same area. These data demonstrate that ZIKV caused febrile disease in NHPs and could be isolated from mosquitoes, solidifying it as an arbovirus [1]. In the years since, many additional isolates have been made and the ones discussed in this review are listed in **Table 1**.

Prior to the major outbreaks in the 2000s, ZIKV had not been detected in the Americas and reported human cases of ZIKV-caused disease were scarce worldwide. Seroprevalence studies in Asia and Africa revealed human populations were exposed to the virus but disease was rarely reported, likely due to a high percentage of asymptomatic infection or because the signs and symptoms were indistinguishable from other known diseases [2]. Data collected during recent outbreaks in Yap Island and across the Americas revealed ZIKV is usually asymptomatic, with symptomatic cases being characterized by flu-like symptoms including self-limiting fever, headache, rash, and myalgia [3].

Worldwide outbreaks in Gabon, Micronesia and French Polynesia expanded the virus' known range and susceptible population, allowing prospective epidemiological studies. ZIKV likely arrived in the Americas in 2014, and in 2015 it quickly spread, starting its largest outbreaks to date [4, 5]. The large number of infected patients and heightened medical and scientific response allowed rare outcomes and transmission routes to be noticed. It was possible to identify that ZIKV causes congenital malformations [6]. Prior to this, cases of miscarriage, microcephaly and other congenital malformations, such as microcephaly or damage to brain and eye tissues, had been identified and were retrospectively observed to be correlated with infection [7, 8]. Infected travelers returning home initiated small traveler-associated transmission cycles, some of which were between sexual partners. Sexual transmission was proposed by Foy and colleagues, who described a probable case of ZIKV sexual transmission of a scientist that visited Senegal in 2008 [9]. Many more cases of sexual transmission were reported after the outbreaks in the Americas, confirming that sexual transmission played a role in the spread of ZIKV, although the full impact of sexual transmission may be underappreciated since it occurs concomitantly with the more efficient transmission by mosquito vectors [10–13].

ZIKV or viral RNA was found to persist in human semen, vaginal secretions and blood [14, 15]. Acquiring samples to study viral persistence in these tissues is difficult because ZIKV infection is frequently asymptomatic and identification of ZIKV-positive samples has to be done by serology or molecular biology, since other viruses that cause similar signs and symptoms are present in the same regions as

Strain	Year Isolation	Lineage	Location	Notes
MR766	1947	African	Ziika forest, Uganda	Contemporaneously available strains are heavily passaged in mice, altering their virulence
PRVABC59	2015	Asian (American)	Puerto Rico	Isolated from human serum during the American outbreak
FSS13025	2010	Asian	French Polynesia	Common isolate used collected prior to the American outbreak. Human isolate
IBH30656	1968	African	Nigeria	Isolated from human blood sample
H/PF/2013	2013	Asian	French Polynesia	Human isolate
BeH815744	2015	Asian (American)	Brazil	Human isolate

Table 1.
Commonly used ZIKV strains.

ZIKV. In Brazil, for example, there are several other flaviviruses and alphaviruses in circulation which produce clinical pictures that cannot be readily differentiated from the signs and symptoms associated with ZIKV. Therefore, molecular and serological tools are critical for the identification and classification of such samples [16]. In many locations, this requires a concerted collaborative effort between hospitals and laboratories, and many samples may need to be shipped before determining which patients came in contact with ZIKV. Additionally, sample collection is made difficult because once symptoms have rescinded, sample collections can no longer be made by hospitals and people may be opposed to having samples collected from them when they are no longer in need of medical care. In spite of these obstacles, several studies were able to assess ZIKV persistence in human samples. In semen, ZIKV RNA was detected for up to 6 months and ZIKV infectious particles could be isolated up to 1 month after primary infection [17]. Vaginal secretions were also found to be positive for RNA for up to 6 months after onset of symptoms [18]. These observations suggest sexual transmission could potentially happen even long after resolution of primary infection. Caution must be taken when trying to directly interpret the consequences of persistent viral RNA since this does not directly imply infectious viral particles. Regardless, transmission is possible, as demonstrated by a woman infecting her partner 44 days after onset of symptoms [13]. Although sexual transmission has most often been reported from males to females, there have been reports of suspected male-to-female [19], male-to-male [20] and female-to-male [21] transmissions. The actual rate of sexual transmission remains unknown.

Our current knowledge of the potential for sexual transmission among members of the *Flavivirus* genus is scarce but it appears that ZIKV is unique among this genus since most members are transmitted between hematophagous arthropods and vertebrate hosts. Although there is limited evidence that other flaviviruses could be sexually transmitted and persist in semen, the currently available body of data does not support this mode of transmission as significant for the spread of these viruses. West Nile virus (WNV) was proposed to have been possibly sexually transmitted in a clinical study of a woman who developed meningo-encephalitis by WNV 2 weeks after intercourse with an infected individual [22]. Other medically important flaviviruses, dengue virus (DENV) [23] and yellow fever virus (YFV) [24], have both been detected in human semen. DENV RNA was detected in a man returning from Thailand to Italy at 37 days post onset of symptoms, when virus RNA was not detectable in the serum or urine anymore [23]. Detection of DENV RNA in the seminal fluid is nevertheless not commonly reported, and another study that performed PCR in the semen of five man with acute DENV infection failed to detect any viral RNA [25]. YFV RNA was detected in urine and semen, but not in the serum, and the virus was isolated from urine on day 21 post onset the symptoms [24]. Another flavivirus, Japanese encephalitis virus (JEV), can be naturally found in porcine semen [26]. JEV was isolated from aborted fetus and semen of pigs which were naturally infected in China from 2004 to 2009 [27]. This raises the question of whether JEV also has the potential to reside in human testes and semen. Experimental approaches have also been used to determine the potential of flaviviruses to be sexually transmitted. Spondweni virus, a close relative to ZIKV, was detected in semen of mice lacking types I and III interferon (AG129) that were inoculated subcutaneously, although this was a rare occurrence when compared to ZIKV-infected AG129 mice [28]. Despite these clinical and experimental reports, the extent of the contribution of sexual transmission to the spread and maintenance of ZIKV in the human population remains unknown.

Examples of sexual transmission may be more common in the family *Flaviviridae* than in the genus *Flavivirus*, as exemplified by bovine viral diarrhea virus (pestivirus, BVDV) in cattle and hepatitis C virus (hepacivirus, HCV) in humans. Both of these infections can cause persistent infections in their hosts under certain conditions and can be sexually transmitted. For BVDV, persistent infection was found in the testes, and bulls persistently shed viral particles in the seminal fluid which allows for sexual transmission [29–31]. For HCV, sexual transmission has been well-documented [32–35]; however, transmission is relatively inefficient [36] and increases with the number of partners, among human immunodeficient virus-positive (HIV+) individuals or among men who have sex with other men [37, 38]. Although there are similarities between ZIKV and these two viruses, caution must be exercised when drawing comparisons, especially when looking for viral determinants of persistence since there are multiple and substantial genomic differences between flaviviruses, pestiviruses and hepaciviruses.

The fact that ZIKV was shown to be sexually transmitted raised many questions, as many aspects of this mode of transmission are poorly understood for these viruses. Namely, the importance of sexual transmission for ZIKV in different regions of the world, the role of cells of the reproductive tract involved in ZIKV persistence and transmission, mutations in the virus which favor successful sexual transmission, interactions of ZIKV with the immune system in the reproductive tract and molecular interactions between ZIKV and host cells allowing for sexual transmission to take place, are all critical points of study. Although abundant data on human disease was generated during the recent outbreaks, animal experiments are an important tool to answer these questions because they allow controlled and rationally designed experiments which could ultimately lead to the development of new vaccines, therapeutics and prophylactic measures. This review will focus on what is currently known for ZIKV infection in the male reproductive tract.

2. Animal models of sexual transmission

Upon discovery of ZIKV, animal experiments were first conducted by Dick [39]. They found that white mice younger than 2 weeks were susceptible to ZIKV infections via intraperitoneal route, whereas mice older than 2 weeks were only susceptible to intracerebral inoculations [39]. Non-human primates inoculated subcutaneously developed neutralizing antibodies against ZIKV and only one animal presented a slight elevation in temperature [39, 40]. Several decades after this initial study, several other model species were used as animal models for ZIKV, but efforts were mostly focused on mice [41–43] and non-human primates (NHPs) [44–47], with most studies being conducted after the outbreak in the Americas in 2015–2016. The experimental design and analyses should carefully consider the anatomical and physiological differences from the species used to humans as well as confounding factors such as different viral strains and inoculation titer and route.

2.1 Mouse models

Mouse models of sexual transmission for ZIKV initially utilized either interferon receptor deficient mice lacking type I (A129) [41] and or type I and II (AG129) interferon receptors [42]. Other models included interferon responsive mouse strains for which a transient knock-down of interferon response was induced by exogenous treatment with antibody against murine type I interferon receptor of wild-type mice or Rag1$^{-/-}$ mice (lacking both B and T lymphocytes) [48]. Several of these models have demonstrated sexual transmission from needle-inoculated male mice to naive female mice following mating. These studies, coupled with the use of surrogate breeding females from which uteri were gavaged, allowed direct assessment of virus and viral RNA shedding efficiency over time. AG129 males infected with ZIKV strain PRVABC59 were shown to shed infectious virus from 7 to 21 days post infection (dpi). Vasectomized males also were shown to shed virus; however, the magnitude was shown to be significantly lower compared to non-vasectomized males [42]. This finding was consistent with a previous study reporting ZIKV RNA shedding in symptomatic men infected with ZIKV in which vasectomized men shed significantly lower levels of ZIKV RNA [17].

The necessity for the use of mice lacking the ability to respond to interferon is due to the inherent resistance of murine STAT2 from being inhibited by ZIKV NS5 [49]. In contrast, human STAT2 has been demonstrated to be highly susceptible to antagonism by ZIKV NS5 [50]. As such, the subsequent development of humanized STAT2 mice have proven useful as a fully interferon responsive model for which ZIKV can replicate and induce pathogenic responses [51].

2.1.1 Sexual transmission murine models

A number of different models have been developed in order to directly assess sexual transmission Sexual transmission has been modeled via direct intravaginal inoculation. In one model, AG129 male mice euthanized and caudal epididymal lumen (containing sperm) was collected. This suspension was used to inoculate female AG129 mice. In this study, the antioxidant ebselen was used to alleviate testicular pathology caused by ZIKV. Although intravaginally inoculated female AG129 mice with sperm from male mice treated with ebselen demonstrated reduced mortality, sexual transmission was not prevented, as female organs (ovary/fallopian tubes, spleen and brain) were infected [52]. Other studies have used homogenized accessory gland fluid and epididymal lumen fluid from Ifnar1$^{-/-}$ male mice subcutaneously inoculated with PRVABC59 to intravaginally inoculated female AG129 mice. In this study, females became viremic and succumbed to infection. Furthermore, progesterone pre-treatment of female mice before intravaginal inoculation was shown to increase mortality of females [53]. IFNAR1$^{-/-}$ male mice inoculated subcutaneously with PRVABC59 and then at 14 dpi or 35 dpi, prostatic and seminal vesicular homogenates and epididymal flushes were collected. Female AG129 mice inoculated intravaginally with this insemination fluid failed to become viremic [54].

Intravaginal inoculation of di-estrus timed AG129 mice or LysMCre^{+}IFNAR$^{fl/fl}$ mice (lacking IFNAR in myeloid cells) was shown to result in viremia and virus replication in peripheral organs and in the vaginal tissues measured by viral assay by RT-PCR through 10 dpi [55]. In an alternative study, immunocompetent C57BL/6 N female mice intravaginally inoculated with PRVABC59 showed a slight increase in viral RNA in the lower female reproductive tract (LFRT) from dpi 1 to 2 and mRNA expression of type I and III IFNs, IRF3/7, RIG-I, and MDA-5 was comparable to uninfected controls, suggesting that a dampened antiviral immune response occurs in the LFRT in response to infection with ZIKV. When mice were treated with an enhancer of RIG-1 signaling, the increase in ZIKV RNA in LFRT was not observed [56]. After intravaginal inoculation during the diestrus phase, ZIKV was shown to replicate in vaginal mucosa of wild type (WT) C57BL/6 and Ifnar1$^{-/-}$ mice. Fetuses from pregnant WT C57BL/6 mice developed intrauterine growth restriction and fetal brains were infected following intravaginal ZIKV inoculation. Fetuses from pregnant IFNAR1$^{-/-}$ mice developed severe intrauterine growth restriction and fetal death was observed. The pregnant females were found to develop viremia. These data are suggestive of an ascending infection from the vaginal tissues to the uterus for fetal involvement [57].

In addition to sexual transmission models that have utilized intravaginal exposure to model sexual transmission potential, several studies have addressed transmission dynamics through direct coitus models. AG129 males were found to sexually transmit to naïve AG129 females in 50% of all matings as measured by subsequent viremias in mated females. This initial study demonstrated *in utero* infection after sexual transmission [42]. A subsequent study compared sexual transmission with subcutaneous and intravaginal routes on female disease presentation, tropism and fetal infection. Sexual transmission of ZIKV to naïve female AG129 mice increased morbidity and mortality in these females as compared to female mice subcutaneously or intravaginally inoculated. Fetuses from females infected via sexual transmission had higher ZIKV titers compared to fetuses from pregnant females infected subcutaneously or intravaginally [58].

2.1.2 Potential sources of sexually transmitted virus/ZIKV infection of the murine testes and epididymides

The majority of ZIKV detected in the seminal fluid of infected AG129 mice during the peak timing of sexual transmission (10–12 dpi) was from the supernatant fraction, suggesting cell-free ZIKV may be largely responsible for sexual transmission. In this study, the testes and epididymides were determined to be infected concurrently and epididymal epithelial cells were identified as the predominant cell population infected in epididymides and shown to contain replicating ZIKV by *in situ* hybridization. In the testes, interstitial leukocytes and peritubular myoid cells were found to be infected initially, followed by extensive infection of all layers of the seminiferous tubule epithelium [59]. Similar results were also shown in IFNAR1$^{-/-}$ mice for which epithelial components of epididymides were identified to be infected and that testes and epididymides could be infected concurrently [60]. In another experiment with immune competent C57BL/6 mice treated with anti-IFNAR1 blocking antibody and subcutaneously inoculated with Asian and African genotype ZIKVs, sexual transmission potential was observed for all viruses with infectious virus identified in the epididymides from all groups even when infectious virus was absent from the testes and seminal vesicles. Infection of the epididymides was demonstrated to be critical for establishing sexual transmission potential, as infectious virus and viral RNA was detected in the epididymides and in semen days before infectious virus was detected in the seminal vesicles or testes [61].

Tissue restricted ZIKVs generated through the incorporation of microRNA target sequences within recombinant ZIKVs were utilized to assess the importance of different cell populations for sexual transmission potential. Testes-restricted ZIKVs could still infect the epididymides, demonstrating a hematogenous/lymphogenous route of infection. Epididymides-restricted ZIKV had high titers in epididymides by plaque assay, but immunohistochemical analysis confirmed epididymides-restricted ZIKV did not replicate in the epididymal epithelium, suggesting that ZIKV is transported from testes to epididymides via excurrent ducts in a cell-free form or transported in sloughed spermatids/infected luminal leukocytes, and ZIKV can infect the epididymides via hematogenous/lymphogenous route of infection [62].

2.1.3 Persistence and tropism of ZIKV on the male reproductive tract

Tropism and persistence of ZIKV in the male reproductive tract may be the key factor responsible for the presence of the virus in semen even long after initial infection. A model of the male mouse reproductive tract is shown in **Figure 1A**. Based on *in vivo* studies, ZIKV is thought to infect the testes, an immunologically privileged site, via a hematogenous route [62] and by infecting the Sertoli cells (SC, **Figure 1B**), an important cell population responsible for the formation of the blood-testes barrier, as shown using AG129 mouse models [63, 64]. SC are critical for spermatogenesis, since they nourish germ cells and help them mature. Tight junctions formed by adjacent SC are functional components of the blood-testes barrier (**Figure 1C**), which prevents molecules from passing between the blood and the lumen of a seminiferous tubule. From the testes, ZIKV can then reach the epididymides by the excurrent testicular route either by infecting germ cells or as free virus particles [62]. ZIKV can also infect the epididymides directly from the hematogenous route [62] (**Figure 1**), and infection of epididymides was observed to happen concurrently with testes infection, indicating that epididymal infection could happen directly and through the testes, or independently of the testes. Infection of germ cells in the testes is not a requirement for sexual transmission as there are reported cases of ZIKV sexual transmission from vasectomized men [65] and in experiments with vasectomized AG129s [42]. Instead, AG129 mouse models indicate that infection of epididymal epithelial cells may the major factor leading to shedding of virus particles in the semen, with these cells being the predominant source of cell-free ZIKV in the seminal fluid [66].

Intracellular viral persistence is likely an important component for long-term sexual transmission. Although the cells that act as reservoirs of ZIKV in testes and the reproductive tract are unknown, possible reservoirs in the host are SC [67, 68] germ cells [69], Leydig cells [70] and epididymal epithelial cells [59, 62] which have been shown to support persistent infections of ZIKV (**Figure 1**). When primary SCs persistently infected with two strains of ZIKV (PRVABC59 or MR766) were monitored for a period of 6 weeks, it was found that 15% of the cells were still positive for both strains of ZIKV [67]. In this same study, Leydig cells were not observed to support persistence [67]. The mechanisms underlying persistence of ZIKV in testes are likely multifactorial and represent a complex phenomenon involving interactions between viral and host factors that needs to be studied in depth. The interactions that occur between ZIKV and host factors that are required for long-term infection of the testes/epididymides are poorly understood and viral persistence likely requires a balance between efficient viral replication and damage caused to host cells. The AXL receptor tyrosine kinase, which was previously shown to be required for entry of ZIKV and other flaviviruses into certain cell types, has been shown to be required for ZIKV entry in SCs [71], but may also be involved in negatively regulating SCs innate immune response [72]. ZIKV infection of SCs results in gene expression changes, with upregulation of antiviral pathways, dysregulation of junction and growth pathways [67, 73]. Although the immune

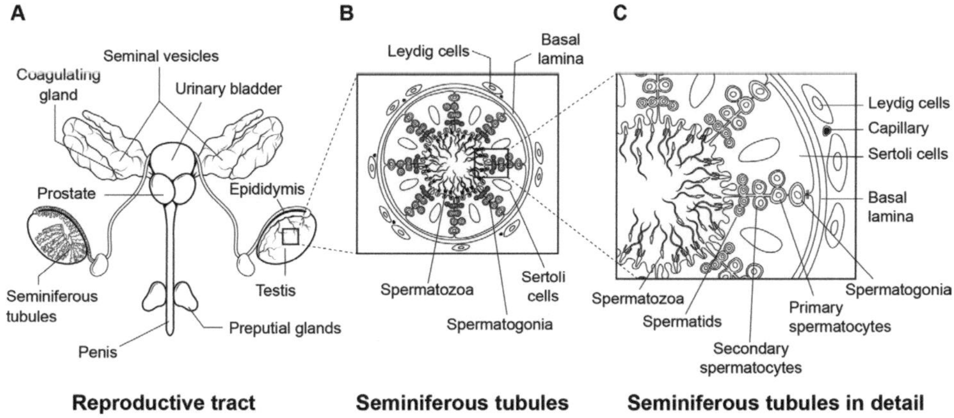

Figure 1.
The male reproductive tract. (A) Overall representation of the male reproductive tract. (B) Seminiferous tubules. (C) Seminiferous tubules in detail.

system of the reproductive tract in females is able to eventually clear ZIKV, largely due to interferon signaling [74, 75], such as the type III interferon lambda [76], the microenvironment of the male testes is an immune-privileged site that lacks adequate response for clearance [77].

2.1.4 Viral genetic changes associated with persistence

Mosquito-vectored flaviviruses that can result in persistent infections are usually associated with an accumulation of adaptive mutations, suggesting that viral genetics may also play an important role for establishing persistence. Examples of mutations in viruses causing persistence were shown with ZIKV, WNV [78–80], JEV [81], YFV [24, 82], and DENV [23]. These mutations happen in different viral proteins and appear to affect various viral functions, but in general attenuate the virus to cause less cytopathic effects, which is likely important for persistence. Identifying the mutations and cellular components that allow flaviviruses to cause long-term infections may elucidate mechanisms by which ZIKV is able to remain stable in seminal fluid long after infection. Although functional mutations in ZIKV may have been found in the male reproductive tract and ejaculates of mice [83], these were do not appear to be specific to these tissues as they were also found after passaging in Vero cells [83], and no mutation has been identified to be required for persistence and/or sexual transmission. Continuing research efforts using animal models are paramount to understand the mechanisms of ZIKV persistence, sexual transmission, reservoirs and interactions with cellular targets.

2.2 Non-human primate (NHP) models

NHP models are also frequently used to study ZIKV since their biology more closely relates to a human than does mouse biology. Several non-human primates were shown to be susceptible to ZIKV and used to study pathogenesis and infection of the reproductive tract, including cynomolgus macaques (*Macaca fascicularis*), rhesus macaques (*Macaca mulatta*), pigtail macaques (*Macaca nemestrina*) and olive baboon (*Papio anubis*), as well as neotropical non-human primates of the *Callithrix, Saimiri and Aotus* genera [46, 84]. These species presented viremia and variable degrees of clinical signs following ZIKV infection. Although many studies were conducted looking at ZIKV pathogenesis and the effects of infection on reproductive tissues, studies directly testing sexual transmission are lacking due to technical and logistical difficulties. Instead, vaginal or rectal inoculations have been used to simulate a sexual transmission. These and other insights into sexual transmission of non-human primates can also shed light on whether this type of transmission play a role in maintenance of ZIKV in nature, since primates are putative ZIKV reservoirs.

Because NHPs are evolutionarily close to humans, it is not surprising that these animals and their reproductive tract are anatomically and physiologically more similar to humans than other models such as mice; thus, NHPs are often considered to be one of the most relevant animal models [85, 86]. Unlike mice, immunocompetent NHPs are more suitable to study ZIKV infections, although the extent to which disease is mimicked is difficult to assess and varies with NHP species. Most NHP models were similar to humans in that most infections were asymptomatic, with clinical signs observed in some individuals [87, 88]. Considering that many human infections are asymptomatic, it is currently unclear if the clinical signs displayed by NHPs are a good model for disease rate and severity in humans. In a study using four cynomolgus macaques one individual was shown to present reduced body temperature [87]. Studying ZIKV pathogenesis in NHPs is important to understand disease progression, clinical signs, negative effects to the reproductive tract and outcomes of pregnancy. These data also inform the design of sexual transmission studies as far as titers, timepoints and strain used for infection, tissues that are important for disease and persistence so sexual transmission can take place. It is worth noting that these experimental infections are performed using virus in a needle while most [89] natural infections occur by a mosquito bite; mosquito saliva has immunomodulatory properties that have been shown to enhance disease in other flaviviral infection [90–92] and could be another confounding factor in these studies.

2.2.1 *Cynomolgus macaque*

Cynomolgus macaques were shown to be suitable as models for ZIKV pathogenesis and sexual transmission [87, 88, 93]. Infection with 5 $\log_{10}$ of plaque forming units (PFU) of ZIKV from various geographical origins resulted in viremia which peaked at 2-4 dpi at 4-7 $\log_{10}$ ZIKV genome copies/ml [87, 88]. The outbreak strain PRVABC59 was more virulent than the Asian FSS13025 and the African IBH30656 ZIKV, with the animals infected with the PRVABC59 strain being viremic for extended periods of time. Bodily fluids checked did not include seminal fluid, and shedding of virus in the urine and saliva was not observed with either the FSS13025 [87] or IBH30656 strains. ZIKV FSS13025 was detected in testes [88], consistent with murine infections with this strain [41]. On the other hand, ZIKV PRVABC59 was detected in urine, saliva and testes [88]. The fact that virus was found in testes suggests this species of NHP could model virus persistence in testes well and may also be a positive feature of this model for sexual transmission in general. The cynomolgus macaque model has also been shown to likely support sexual transmission, as macaques inoculated with 7 $\log_{10}$ PFU of virus intravaginally and intrarectally became viremic 50% and 100% of the time, respectively [93]. To understand the implications of these findings would be important to know the ranges of ZIKV titers in the semen. Although it is not clear what the viral titers are in most human semen samples, studies detected up to 9 $\log_{10}$ RNA copies/ml of virus in semen of patients [17, 89].

2.2.2 *Olive baboon*

As with cynomolgus macaques, infection of olive baboons with different strains of ZIKV did not result in overt clinical signs. Following subcutaneous inoculation of a French Polynesian ZIKV (H/PF/2013), the baboons presented viremia that peaked at 3 and 4 dpi [45]. Around 40 days post infection, tissues were collected and virus was found in lymph nodes and epididymides, suggesting these are the places where the virus can persist even after viral clearance from the blood [45]. This suggests the testes were likely infected at some point and that the epididymides may also play a role in virus persistence [45]. Olive baboons were also used to model ZIKV infection during pregnancy. Infection of 4 $\log_{10}$ of ZIKV H/PF/2013 resulted in vertical transmission in 3 out of 4 pregnant NHPs [94]. Unlike the non-pregnant animals, all dams presented rash and conjunctivitis [94]. Fetal death and defects in the frontal cortex of the fetus were observed [94].

2.2.3 *Rhesus macaque*

The rhesus macaque is perhaps the most utilized NHP model to study ZIKV infection. Many studies of ZIKV were done using this species, including pathogenesis analyses in pregnant and non-pregnant animals, immunological and serological studies, and testing of anti-ZIKV vaccines or drugs [44, 95–106]. A study in which ZIKV was inoculated intravaginally in rhesus macaques to mimic sexual transmission found ZIKV RNA in the reproductive tract of all 6 animals infected, thus raising the question of whether fetal disease could be more pronounced after sexual transmission when compared to vectored transmission [103]. This study lacked subcutaneous inoculation controls and further studies need to be conducted to confirm these findings. Another study comparing the intravaginal and subcutaneous routes using ZIKV PRVABC59 found peak viremia at 5–8 dpi that were variable in titer (3–7.5 $\log_{10}$ PFUs). Although the types of tissue found to be positive differed between subcutaneous and intravaginal inoculated animals, there was no obvious preference for reproductive tract tissues in the intravaginal route [107]. The data showed that intravaginal infection resulted in less $CD11C^{hi}$ myeloid cells, reduced expression of programmed cell death protein 1 (PD-1) in natural killer cells (NK) and more Ki67+ CD8+ central memory cells, indicating the route of infection may play a role in shaping the immune response [107].

Persistent ZIKV in reproductive tissues may play a role in sexual transmission long after primary infection. After intravenous inoculation of 5 $\log_{10}$ of a Brazilian ZIKV (BeH815744) in female rhesus macaques, ZIKV RNA was detected in multiple tissues of the NHPs, including reproductive tissues 14 dpi [108]. Lymphoid tissues had the highest detectable amount of viral RNA, suggesting these organs, which span many parts of the body, may act as possible viral reservoir [108].

2.3 Other animal models

Several other animal models have been used to study ZIKV but most are not focused on sexual transmission. These models include guinea pigs [109–111], hamsters [112], bats [113], chick embryos, piglets [114, 115] and boars [116]. Porcine fetuses were shown to present mild to severe neuropathology upon ZIKV infection [114, 115]. Boar semen was inoculated with ZIKV, but it was concluded that ZIKV does not appear to cause cell damage and cannot replicate efficiently or persist in the semen of this species [116]. With respect to the neotropical chiropteran model, viral RNA was found in different tissues of fruit bats 28 dpi, suggesting ZIKV can infect bats which may serve as virus reservoirs. Bats did not show any signs of disease [113]. Stat-2 knockout hamsters infected with ZIKV have shown presence on infected cells with morphology of SCs and spermatogonia, suggesting this could be a suitable model to study persistence of the virus in testes [112]. The guinea pig models report conflicting results. One study with ZIKV challenge mid-gestation showed no evidence of infection [109]; however, Kumar et al. show guinea pigs inoculated subcutaneously with PRVABC59 had viremia and presented signs such as fever, hunched posture and detectable viral RNA in the blood [110]. Deng et al. showed that intranasally-infected guinea pigs have virus in the sera, saliva and tears [111].

3. Conclusions

ZIKV has emerged explosively since 2007, causing an epidemic in the Americas in 2015/16 and become a matter of global health importance. Although data from epidemiologic analyses and case studies helped shed light on the diseases caused by ZIKV, animal models will be important to substantiate and extend these findings under controlled experimental settings. Animal models can be—and have already proven to be—useful as a tool to understand ZIKV transmission and ZIKV-caused illnesses. Animal models do not fully recapitulate diseases as seen in humans; therefore, it is critical to consider the advantages and drawbacks of each model when designing and executing the experiments as well as interpreting the data. Models to study sexual transmission are currently scarce and need further development. Challenges include scarcity of good models to study ZIKV sexual transmission, low number of animals used and the requirement to improve reproducibility of the findings from animal models, which is caused by differences in experimental conditions and the number of animals used. As in certain cases increasing the number of animals used is not possible due to it being prohibitively expensive or posing ethical issues, future experiments assessing sexual transmission of ZIKV should focus on optimizing experimental design and analysis, when possible standardizing experimental conditions so they can be compared between studies.

Acknowledgements

We thank Drs. Sasha Azar and Nikos Vasilakis for their critical reading of the chapter and helpful discussions.

Conflict of interest

We have no conflicts of interest to declare.

Author details

Rafael K. Campos[1], Erin M. McDonald[2], Aaron C. Brault[2*] and Shannan L. Rossi[1*]

1 Department of Microbiology and Immunology, University of Texas Medical Branch, Galveston, USA

2 Division of Vector-Borne Diseases, National Center for Emerging and Zoonotic Infectious Diseases (NCEZID), Centers for Disease Control and Prevention (CDC), USA

*Address all correspondence to: zlu5@cdc.gov and slrossi@utmb.edu

References

[1] Dick GW, Kitchen SF, Haddow AJ. Zika virus. I. Isolations and serological specificity. Transactions of the Royal Society of Tropical Medicine and Hygiene. 1952;**46**(5):509-520

[2] Haddow AD, Schuh AJ, Yasuda CY, Kasper MR, Heang V, Huy R, et al. Genetic characterization of Zika virus strains: Geographic expansion of the Asian lineage. PLoS Neglected Tropical Diseases. 2012;**6**(2):e1477

[3] Musso D, Gubler DJ. Zika virus. Clinical Microbiology Reviews. 2016;**29**(3):487-524

[4] Weaver SC, Costa F, Garcia-Blanco MA, Ko AI, Ribeiro GS, Saade G, et al. Zika virus: History, emergence, biology, and prospects for control. Antiviral Research. 2016;**130**:69-80

[5] Campos GS, Bandeira AC, Sardi SI. Zika virus outbreak, Bahia, Brazil. Emerging Infectious Diseases. 2015;**21**(10):1885-1886

[6] Ventura CV, Maia M, Bravo-Filho V, Gois AL, Belfort R Jr. Zika virus in Brazil and macular atrophy in a child with microcephaly. Lancet. 2016;**387**(10015):228

[7] van der Eijk AA, van Genderen PJ, Verdijk RM, Reusken CB, Mogling R, van Kampen JJ, et al. Miscarriage associated with Zika virus infection. The New England Journal of Medicine. 2016;**375**(10):1002-1004

[8] Cauchemez S, Besnard M, Bompard P, Dub T, Guillemette-Artur P, Eyrolle-Guignot D, et al. Association between Zika virus and microcephaly in French Polynesia, 2013-15: A retrospective study. Lancet. 2016;**387**(10033):2125-2132

[9] Foy BD, Kobylinski KC, Chilson Foy JL, Blitvich BJ, Travassos da Rosa A, Haddow AD, et al. Probable non-vector-borne transmission of Zika virus, Colorado, USA. Emerging Infectious Diseases. 2011;**17**(5):880-882

[10] Musso D, Roche C, Robin E, Nhan T, Teissier A, Cao-Lormeau VM. Potential sexual transmission of Zika virus. Emerging Infectious Diseases. 2015;**21**(2):359-361

[11] D'Ortenzio E, Matheron S, Yazdanpanah Y, de Lamballerie X, Hubert B, Piorkowski G, et al. Evidence of sexual transmission of Zika virus. The New England Journal of Medicine. 2016;**374**(22):2195-2198

[12] Freour T, Mirallie S, Hubert B, Splingart C, Barriere P, Maquart M, et al. Sexual transmission of Zika virus in an entirely asymptomatic couple returning from a Zika epidemic area, France, April 2016. Euro Surveillance: Bulletin Europeen sur les Maladies Transmissibles = European Communicable Disease Bulletin. 2016;**21**(23):30254

[13] Turmel JM, Abgueguen P, Hubert B, Vandamme YM, Maquart M, Le Guillou-Guillemette H, et al. Late sexual transmission of Zika virus related to persistence in the semen. Lancet. 2016;**387**(10037):2501

[14] Aliota MT, Bassit L, Bradrick SS, Cox B, Garcia-Blanco MA, Gavegnano C, et al. Zika in the Americas, year 2: What have we learned? What gaps remain? A report from the Global Virus Network. Antiviral Research. 2017;**144**:223-246

[15] Prisant N, Bujan L, Benichou H, Hayot PH, Pavili L, Lurel S, et al. Zika virus in the female genital tract. The Lancet Infectious Diseases. 2016;**16**(9):1000-1001

[16] Waggoner JJ, Pinsky BA. Zika virus: Diagnostics for an emerging pandemic

threat. Journal of Clinical Microbiology. 2016;**54**(4):860-867

[17] Mead PS, Duggal NK, Hook SA, Delorey M, Fischer M, Olzenak McGuire D, et al. Zika virus shedding in semen of symptomatic infected men. The New England Journal of Medicine. 2018;**378**(15):1377-1385

[18] Reyes Y, Bowman NM, Becker-Dreps S, Centeno E, Collins MH, Liou GA, et al. Prolonged shedding of Zika virus RNA in vaginal secretions, Nicaragua. Emerging Infectious Diseases. 2019;**25**(4):808-810

[19] Russell K, Hills SL, Oster AM, Porse CC, Danyluk G, Cone M, et al. Male-to-female sexual transmission of Zika virus-United States, January-April 2016. Clinical Infectious Diseases. 2017;**64**(2):211-213

[20] Deckard DT, Chung WM, Brooks JT, Smith JC, Woldai S, Hennessey M, et al. Male-to-male sexual transmission of Zika virus—Texas, January 2016. MMWR. Morbidity and Mortality Weekly Report. 2016;**65**(14):372-374

[21] Davidson A, Slavinski S, Komoto K, Rakeman J, Weiss D. Suspected female-to-male sexual transmission of Zika virus—New York City, 2016. MMWR. Morbidity and Mortality Weekly Report. 2016;**65**(28):716-717

[22] Kelley RE, Berger JR, Kelley BP. West Nile virus Meningo-encephalitis: Possible sexual transmission. Journal of the Louisiana State Medical Society. 2016;**168**(1):21-22

[23] Lalle E, Colavita F, Iannetta M, Gebremeskel Tekle S, Carletti F, Scorzolini L, et al. Prolonged detection of dengue virus RNA in the semen of a man returning from Thailand to Italy, January 2018. Euro Surveillance: Bulletin Europeen sur les Maladies Transmissibles = European Communicable Disease Bulletin. 2018;**23**(18):18-00197

[24] Barbosa CM, Di Paola N, Cunha MP, Rodrigues-Jesus MJ, Araujo DB, Silveira VB, et al. Yellow fever virus RNA in urine and semen of convalescent patient, Brazil. Emerging Infectious Diseases. 2018;**24**(1):176-178

[25] Molton JS, Low I, Choy MMJ, Aw PPK, Hibberd ML, Tambyah PA, et al. Dengue virus not detected in human semen. Journal of Travel Medicine. 2018;**25**(1):1-3

[26] Althouse GC, Rossow K. The potential risk of infectious disease dissemination via artificial insemination in swine. Reproduction in Domestic Animals. 2011;**46**(Suppl 2):64-67

[27] Liu WJ, Zhu M, Pei JJ, Dong XY, Liu W, Zhao MQ, et al. Molecular phylogenetic and positive selection analysis of Japanese encephalitis virus strains isolated from pigs in China. Virus Research. 2013;**178**(2):547-552

[28] McDonald EM, Duggal NK, Brault AC. Pathogenesis and sexual transmission of Spondweni and Zika viruses. PLoS Neglected Tropical Diseases. 2017;**11**(10):e0005990

[29] Rikula U, Nuotio L, Laamanen UI, Sihvonen L. Transmission of bovine viral diarrhoea virus through the semen of acutely infected bulls under field conditions. The Veterinary Record. 2008;**162**(3):79-82

[30] Newcomer BW, Toohey-Kurth K, Zhang Y, Brodersen BW, Marley MS, Joiner KS, et al. Laboratory diagnosis and transmissibility of bovine viral diarrhea virus from a bull with a persistent testicular infection. Veterinary Microbiology. 2014;**170**(3-4):246-257

[31] Voges H, Horner GW, Rowe S, Wellenberg GJ. Persistent bovine

pestivirus infection localized in the testes of an immuno-competent, non-viraemic bull. Veterinary Microbiology. 1998;**61**(3):165-175

[32] Sanchez-Quijano A, Rey C, Aguado I, Pineda JA, Perez-Romero M, Torres Y, et al. Hepatitis C virus infection in sexually promiscuous groups. European Journal of Clinical Microbiology & Infectious Diseases. 1990;**9**(8):610-612

[33] Salvaggio A, Conti M, Albano A, Pianetti A, Muggiasca ML, Re M, et al. Sexual transmission of hepatitis C virus and HIV-1 infection in female intravenous drug users. European Journal of Epidemiology. 1993;**9**(3):279-284

[34] Leruez-Ville M, Kunstmann JM, De Almeida M, Rouzioux C, Chaix ML. Detection of hepatitis C virus in the semen of infected men. Lancet. 2000;**356**(9223):42-43

[35] Sanchez-Beiza L, Bravo R, Toribio R, Navarro S, Soriano V. Sexual transmission of two different HCV types causing acute hepatitis C. Vox Sanguinis. 1996;**71**(4):244-245

[36] Marincovich B, Castilla J, del Romero J, Garcia S, Hernando V, Raposo M, et al. Absence of hepatitis C virus transmission in a prospective cohort of heterosexual serodiscordant couples. Sexually Transmitted Infections. 2003;**79**(2):160-162

[37] van de Laar TJ, van der Bij AK, Prins M, Bruisten SM, Brinkman K, Ruys TA, et al. Increase in HCV incidence among men who have sex with men in Amsterdam most likely caused by sexual transmission. The Journal of Infectious Diseases. 2007;**196**(2):230-238

[38] Dienstag JL. Sexual and perinatal transmission of hepatitis C. Hepatology. 1997;**26**(3 Suppl 1):66S-70S

[39] Dick GW. Zika virus. II. Pathogenicity and physical properties. Transactions of the Royal Society of Tropical Medicine and Hygiene. 1952;**46**(5):521-534

[40] Taylor RM. Studies on certain viruses isolated in the tropics of Africa and South America; their growth and behavior in the embryonated hen egg. Journal of Immunology. 1952;**68**(4):473-494

[41] Rossi SL, Tesh RB, Azar SR, Muruato AE, Hanley KA, Auguste AJ, et al. Characterization of a novel murine model to study Zika virus. The American Journal of Tropical Medicine and Hygiene. 2016;**94**(6):1362-1369

[42] Duggal NK, Ritter JM, Pestorius SE, Zaki SR, Davis BS, Chang GJ, et al. Frequent Zika virus sexual transmission and prolonged viral RNA shedding in an Immunodeficient mouse model. Cell Reports. 2017;**18**(7):1751-1760

[43] Lazear HM, Govero J, Smith AM, Platt DJ, Fernandez E, Miner JJ, et al. A mouse model of Zika virus pathogenesis. Cell Host & Microbe. 2016;**19**(5):720-730

[44] Dudley DM, Aliota MT, Mohr EL, Weiler AM, Lehrer-Brey G, Weisgrau KL, et al. A rhesus macaque model of Asian-lineage Zika virus infection. Nature Communications. 2016;**7**:12204

[45] Gurung S, Preno AN, Dubaut JP, Nadeau H, Hyatt K, Reuter N, et al. Translational model of Zika virus disease in baboons. Journal of Virology. 2018;**92**(16):e00186-18

[46] Vanchiere JA, Ruiz JC, Brady AG, Kuehl TJ, Williams LE, Baze WB, et al. Experimental Zika virus infection of neotropical primates. The American Journal of Tropical Medicine and Hygiene. 2018;**98**(1):173-177

[47] Osuna CE, Lim SY, Deleage C, Griffin BD, Stein D, Schroeder LT, et al. Zika viral dynamics and shedding in rhesus and cynomolgus macaques. Nature Medicine. 2016;**22**(12):1448-1455

[48] Winkler CW, Myers LM, Woods TA, Messer RJ, Carmody AB, McNally KL, et al. Adaptive immune responses to Zika virus are important for controlling virus infection and preventing infection in brain and testes. Journal of Immunology. 2017;**198**(9):3526-3535

[49] Tripathi S, Balasubramaniam VR, Brown JA, Mena I, Grant A, Bardina SV, et al. A novel Zika virus mouse model reveals strain specific differences in virus pathogenesis and host inflammatory immune responses. PLoS Pathogens. 2017;**13**(3):e1006258

[50] Grant A, Ponia SS, Tripathi S, Balasubramaniam V, Miorin L, Sourisseau M, et al. Zika virus targets human STAT2 to inhibit type I interferon signaling. Cell Host & Microbe. 2016;**19**(6):882-890

[51] Gorman MJ, Caine EA, Zaitsev K, Begley MC, Weger-Lucarelli J, Uccellini MB, et al. An immuno-competent mouse model of Zika virus infection. Cell Host & Microbe. 2018;**23**(5):672-685 e6

[52] Simanjuntak Y, Liang JJ, Chen SY, Li JK, Lee YL, Wu HC, et al. Ebselen alleviates testicular pathology in mice with Zika virus infection and prevents its sexual transmission. PLoS Pathogens. 2018;**14**(2):e1006854

[53] Clancy CS, Van Wettere AJ, Morrey JD, Julander JG. Coitus-free sexual transmission of Zika virus in a mouse model. Scientific Reports. 2018;**8**(1):15379

[54] Clancy CS, Van Wettere AJ, Morrey JD, Julander JG. Zika virus associated pathology and antigen presence in the testicle in the absence of sexual transmission during subacute to chronic infection in a mouse model. Scientific Reports. 2019;**9**(1):8325

[55] Tang WW, Young MP, Mamidi A, Regla-Nava JA, Kim K, Shresta S. A mouse model of Zika virus sexual transmission and vaginal viral replication. Cell Reports. 2016;**17**(12):3091-3098

[56] Khan S, Woodruff EM, Trapecar M, Fontaine KA, Ezaki A, Borbet TC, et al. Dampened antiviral immunity to intravaginal exposure to RNA viral pathogens allows enhanced viral replication. The Journal of Experimental Medicine. 2016;**213**(13):2913-2929

[57] Yockey LJ, Varela L, Rakib T, Khoury-Hanold W, Fink SL, Stutz B, et al. Vaginal exposure to Zika virus during pregnancy leads to fetal brain infection. Cell. 2016;**166**(5): 1247-1256 e4

[58] Duggal NK, McDonald EM, Ritter JM, Brault AC. Sexual transmission of Zika virus enhances in utero transmission in a mouse model. Scientific Reports. 2018;**8**(1):4510

[59] McDonald EM, Duggal NK, Ritter JM, Brault AC. Infection of epididymal epithelial cells and leukocytes drives seminal shedding of Zika virus in a mouse model. PLoS Neglected Tropical Diseases. 2018;**12**(8):e0006691

[60] Clancy CS, Van Wettere AJ, Siddharthan V, Morrey JD, Julander JG. Comparative histopathologic lesions of the male reproductive tract during acute infection of Zika virus in AG129 and Ifnar(−/−) mice. The American Journal of Pathology. 2018;**188**(4):904-915

[61] McDonald EM, Duggal NK, Delorey MJ, Oksanish J, Ritter JM, Brault AC. Duration of seminal Zika viral RNA shedding in immunocompetent mice inoculated with Asian and

African genotype viruses. Virology. 2019;**535**:1-10

[62] Tsetsarkin KA, Maximova OA, Liu G, Kenney H, Teterina N, Bloom ME, et al. Routes of Zika virus dissemination in the testis and epididymis of immunodeficient mice. Nature Communications. 2018;**9**(1):5350

[63] Siemann DN, Strange DP, Maharaj PN, Shi PY, Verma S. Zika virus infects human sertoli cells and modulates the integrity of the in vitro blood-testis barrier model. Journal of Virology. 2017;**91**(22):e00623-17

[64] Sheng ZY, Gao N, Wang ZY, Cui XY, Zhou DS, Fan DY, et al. Sertoli cells are susceptible to ZIKV infection in mouse testis. Frontiers in Cellular and Infection Microbiology. 2017;**7**:272

[65] Arsuaga M, Bujalance SG, Diaz-Menendez M, Vazquez A, Arribas JR. Probable sexual transmission of Zika virus from a vasectomised man. The Lancet Infectious Diseases. 2016;**16**(10):1107

[66] Ma W, Li S, Ma S, Jia L, Zhang F, Zhang Y, et al. Zika virus causes testis damage and leads to male infertility in mice. Cell. 2016;**167**(6):1511-1524 e10

[67] Kumar A, Jovel J, Lopez-Orozco J, Limonta D, Airo AM, Hou S, et al. Human Sertoli cells support high levels of Zika virus replication and persistence. Scientific Reports. 2018;**8**(1):5477

[68] Mlera L, Bloom ME. Differential Zika virus infection of testicular cell lines. Viruses. 2019;**11**(1):E42

[69] Robinson CL, Chong ACN, Ashbrook AW, Jeng G, Jin J, Chen H, et al. Male germ cells support long-term propagation of Zika virus. Nature Communications. 2018;**9**(1):2090

[70] Uraki R, Hwang J, Jurado KA, Householder S, Yockey LJ, Hastings AK, et al. Zika virus causes testicular atrophy. Science Advances. 2017;**3**(2):e1602899

[71] Strange DP, Jiyarom B, Pourhabibi Zarandi N, Xie X, Baker C, Sadri-Ardekani H, et al. Axl promotes Zika virus entry and modulates the antiviral state of human sertoli cells. MBio. 2019;**10**(4):e01372-19

[72] Sun B, Qi N, Shang T, Wu H, Deng T, Han D. Sertoli cell-initiated testicular innate immune response through toll-like receptor-3 activation is negatively regulated by Tyro3, Axl, and mer receptors. Endocrinology. 2010;**151**(6):2886-2897

[73] Strange DP, Green R, Siemann DN, Gale M Jr, Verma S. Immunoprofiles of human Sertoli cells infected with Zika virus reveals unique insights into host-pathogen crosstalk. Scientific Reports. 2018;**8**(1):8702

[74] Fung KY, Mangan NE, Cumming H, Horvat JC, Mayall JR, Stifter SA, et al. Interferon-epsilon protects the female reproductive tract from viral and bacterial infection. Science. 2013;**339**(6123):1088-1092

[75] Cumming HE, Bourke NM. Type I IFNs in the female reproductive tract: The first line of defense in an ever-changing battleground. Journal of Leukocyte Biology. 2019;**105**(2):353-361

[76] Caine EA, Scheaffer SM, Arora N, Zaitsev K, Artyomov MN, Coyne CB, et al. Interferon lambda protects the female reproductive tract against Zika virus infection. Nature Communications. 2019;**10**(1):280

[77] Arevalo Romero H, Vargas Pavia TA, Velazquez Cervantes MA, Flores Pliego A, Helguera Repetto AC, Leon Juarez M. The dual role of the immune

response in reproductive organs during Zika virus infection. Frontiers in Immunology. 2019;**10**:1617

[78] Rossi SL, Zhao Q, O'Donnell VK, Mason PW. Adaptation of West Nile virus replicons to cells in culture and use of replicon-bearing cells to probe antiviral action. Virology. 2005;**331**(2):457-470

[79] Rossi SL, Fayzulin R, Dewsbury N, Bourne N, Mason PW. Mutations in West Nile virus nonstructural proteins that facilitate replicon persistence in vitro attenuate virus replication in vitro and in vivo. Virology. 2007;**364**(1):184-195

[80] Lustig Y, Lanciotti RS, Hindiyeh M, Keller N, Milo R, Mayan S, et al. Mutation in West Nile virus structural protein prM during human infection. Emerging Infectious Diseases. 2016;**22**(9):1647-1649

[81] Lyoo HR, Park SY, Kim JY, Jeong YS. Constant up-regulation of BiP/GRP78 expression prevents virus-induced apoptosis in BHK-21 cells with Japanese encephalitis virus persistent infection. Virology Journal. 2015;**12**:32

[82] Vlaycheva L, Nickells M, Droll DA, Chambers TJ. Yellow fever 17D virus: Pseudo-revertant suppression of defective virus penetration and spread by mutations in domains II and III of the E protein. Virology. 2004;**327**(1):41-49

[83] Duggal NK, McDonald EM, Weger-Lucarelli J, Hawks SA, Ritter JM, Romo H, et al. Mutations present in a low-passage Zika virus isolate result in attenuated pathogenesis in mice. Virology. 2019;**530**:19-26

[84] Terzian ACB, Zini N, Sacchetto L, Rocha RF, Parra MCP, Del Sarto JL, et al. Evidence of natural Zika virus infection in neotropical non-human primates in Brazil. Scientific Reports. 2018;**8**(1):16034

[85] Kerr JB. Functional cytology of the human testis. Baillière's Clinical Endocrinology and Metabolism. 1992;**6**(2):235-250

[86] Fayomi AP, Orwig KE. Spermatogonial stem cells and spermatogenesis in mice, monkeys and men. Stem Cell Research. 2018;**29**:207-214

[87] Azar SR, Rossi SL, Haller SH, Yun R, Huang JH, Plante JA, et al. ZIKV demonstrates minimal pathologic effects and mosquito infectivity in viremic cynomolgus macaques. Viruses. 2018;**10**(11):E661

[88] Koide F, Goebel S, Snyder B, Walters KB, Gast A, Hagelin K, et al. Development of a Zika virus infection model in cynomolgus macaques. Frontiers in Microbiology. 2016;**7**:2028

[89] de Laval F, Matheus S, Labrousse T, Enfissi A, Rousset D, Briolant S. Kinetics of Zika viral load in semen. The New England Journal of Medicine. 2017;**377**(7):697-699

[90] Surasombatpattana P, Patramool S, Luplertlop N, Yssel H, Misse D. Aedes aegypti saliva enhances dengue virus infection of human keratinocytes by suppressing innate immune responses. The Journal of Investigative Dermatology. 2012;**132**(8):2103-2105

[91] Styer LM, Lim PY, Louie KL, Albright RG, Kramer LD, Bernard KA. Mosquito saliva causes enhancement of West Nile virus infection in mice. Journal of Virology. 2011;**85**(4):1517-1527

[92] Schneider BS, Higgs S. The enhancement of arbovirus transmission and disease by mosquito saliva is associated with modulation of the host immune response. Transactions of the Royal Society of Tropical Medicine and Hygiene. 2008;**102**(5):400-408

[93] Haddow AD, Nalca A, Rossi FD, Miller LJ, Wiley MR, Perez-Sautu U, et al. High infection rates for adult macaques after intravaginal or intrarectal inoculation with Zika virus. Emerging Infectious Diseases. 2017;**23**(8):1274-1281

[94] Gurung S, Reuter N, Preno A, Dubaut J, Nadeau H, Hyatt K, et al. Zika virus infection at mid-gestation results in fetal cerebral cortical injury and fetal death in the olive baboon. PLoS Pathogens. 2019;**15**(1):e1007507

[95] Maness NJ, Schouest B, Singapuri A, Dennis M, Gilbert MH, Bohm RP, et al. Postnatal Zika virus infection of nonhuman primate infants born to mothers infected with homologous Brazilian Zika virus. Scientific Reports. 2019;**9**(1):12802

[96] Valiant WG, Mattapallil MJ, Higgs S, Huang YS, Vanlandingham DL, Lewis MG, et al. Simultaneous coinfection of macaques with Zika and dengue viruses does not enhance acute plasma viremia but leads to activation of monocyte subsets and biphasic release of pro-inflammatory cytokines. Scientific Reports. 2019;**9**(1):7877

[97] Bidokhti MRM, Dutta D, Madduri LSV, Woollard SM, Norgren R Jr, Giavedoni L, et al. SIV/SHIV-Zika co-infection does not alter disease pathogenesis in adult non-pregnant rhesus macaque model. PLoS Neglected Tropical Diseases. 2018;**12**(10):e0006811

[98] Coffey LL, Keesler RI, Pesavento PA, Woolard K, Singapuri A, Watanabe J, et al. Intraamniotic Zika virus inoculation of pregnant rhesus macaques produces fetal neurologic disease. Nature Communications. 2018;**9**(1):2414

[99] Mavigner M, Raper J, Kovacs-Balint Z, Gumber S, O'Neal JT, Bhaumik SK, et al. Postnatal Zika virus infection is associated with persistent abnormalities in brain structure, function, and behavior in infant macaques. Science Translational Medicine. 2018;**10**(435):eaao6975

[100] Martinot AJ, Abbink P, Afacan O, Prohl AK, Bronson R, Hecht JL, et al. Fetal neuropathology in Zika virus-infected pregnant female rhesus monkeys. Cell. 2018;**173**(5):1111-1122 e10

[101] Hirsch AJ, Roberts VHJ, Grigsby PL, Haese N, Schabel MC, Wang X, et al. Zika virus infection in pregnant rhesus macaques causes placental dysfunction and immunopathology. Nature Communications. 2018;**9**(1):263

[102] Abbink P, Larocca RA, Visitsunthorn K, Boyd M, De La Barrera RA, Gromowski GD, et al. Durability and correlates of vaccine protection against Zika virus in rhesus monkeys. Science Translational Medicine. 2017;**9**(420):eaao4163

[103] Carroll T, Lo M, Lanteri M, Dutra J, Zarbock K, Silveira P, et al. Zika virus preferentially replicates in the female reproductive tract after vaginal inoculation of rhesus macaques. PLoS Pathogens. 2017;**13**(7):e1006537

[104] Nguyen SM, Antony KM, Dudley DM, Kohn S, Simmons HA, Wolfe B, et al. Highly efficient maternal-fetal Zika virus transmission in pregnant rhesus macaques. PLoS Pathogens. 2017;**13**(5):e1006378

[105] Aliota MT, Dudley DM, Newman CM, Mohr EL, Gellerup DD, Breitbach ME, et al. Heterologous protection against Asian Zika virus challenge in rhesus macaques. PLoS Neglected Tropical Diseases. 2016;**10**(12):e0005168

[106] Best K, Guedj J, Madelain V, de Lamballerie X, Lim SY, Osuna CE, et al.

Zika plasma viral dynamics in nonhuman primates provides insights into early infection and antiviral strategies. Proceedings of the National Academy of Sciences of the United States of America. 2017;**114**(33):8847-8852

[107] Woollard SM, Olwenyi OA, Dutta D, Dave RS, Mathews S, Gorantla S, et al. Preliminary studies on immune response and viral pathogenesis of Zika virus in rhesus macaques. Pathogens. 2018;**7**(3):E70

[108] Coffey LL, Pesavento PA, Keesler RI, Singapuri A, Watanabe J, Watanabe R, et al. Zika virus tissue and blood compartmentalization in acute infection of rhesus macaques. PLoS One. 2017;**12**(1):e0171148

[109] Bierle CJ, Fernandez-Alarcon C, Hernandez-Alvarado N, Zabeli JC, Janus BC, Putri DS, et al. Assessing Zika virus replication and the development of Zika-specific antibodies after a mid-gestation viral challenge in Guinea pigs. PLoS One. 2017;**12**(11):e0187720

[110] Kumar M, Krause KK, Azouz F, Nakano E, Nerurkar VR. A Guinea pig model of Zika virus infection. Virology Journal. 2017;**14**(1):75

[111] Deng YQ, Zhang NN, Li XF, Wang YQ, Tian M, Qiu YF, et al. Intranasal infection and contact transmission of Zika virus in Guinea pigs. Nature Communications. 2017;**8**(1):1648

[112] Siddharthan V, Van Wettere AJ, Li R, Miao J, Wang Z, Morrey JD, et al. Zika virus infection of adult and fetal STAT2 knock-out hamsters. Virology. 2017;**507**:89-95

[113] Malmlov A, Bantle C, Aboellail T, Wagner K, Campbell CL, Eckley M, et al. Experimental Zika virus infection of Jamaican fruit bats (*Artibeus jamaicensis*) and possible entry of virus into brain via activated microglial cells. PLoS Neglected Tropical Diseases. 2019;**13**(2):e0007071

[114] Wichgers Schreur PJ, van Keulen L, Anjema D, Kant J, Kortekaas J. Microencephaly in fetal piglets following in utero inoculation of Zika virus. Emerging Microbes and Infections. 2018;**7**(1):42

[115] Darbellay J, Cox B, Lai K, Delgado-Ortega M, Wheler C, Wilson D, et al. Zika virus causes persistent infection in porcine conceptuses and may impair health in offspring. eBioMedicine. 2017;**25**:73-86

[116] Luplertlop N, Suwanmanee S, Ampawong S, Vongpunsawad S, Poovorawan Y. In vitro study of Zika virus infection in boar semen. Archives of Virology. 2017;**162**(10):3209-3213

Section 2

Clinical Aspects

Chapter 4

Clinical Manifestations in Pregnant Women and Congenital Abnormalities in Fetus and Newborns during a Zika Transmission Period in South Mexico

Norma Pavía-Ruz, Silvina Noemí Contreras-Capetillo, Yamila Romer, Nina Valadez Gonzalez, Hector Gómez-Dantés, Gonzalo Vázquez-Prokopec and Pablo Manrique-Saide

Abstract

Dengue, Chikungunya and Zika are arboviruses transmitted by *Ae. aegypti* with significant public health impact. In the first trimester of 2015, autochthonous Zika transmission was reported in Mexico. The state of Yucatan is an endemic region where pregnant women with acute infection and related congenital abnormalities in fetus and newborns were observed. We describe results from a cohort of pregnant women and their babies followed up in Yucatan during the first Zika transmission outbreak (2016–2018). Clinical manifestations of acute ZIKV infection, persistence of viral RNA in pregnant women, as well as congenital abnormalities were observed. In addition, we describe the phenotype of newborns from confirmed or suspected ZIKV prenatal infection.

Keywords: Zika infection, pregnant women birth defects, pregnancy, congenital Zika syndrome

1. Introduction

Dengue (DEN), Chikungunya (CHIK) and Zika (ZIKV) are arboviruses transmitted by the mosquito *Aedes aegypti* and known as *Aedes*-borne-diseases. These diseases are associated with high morbidity and low mortality and considered a public health problem [1]. In the 2015, the ZIKV outbreak was considered an international emergency because infection in pregnant women was related to the increase of congenital abnormalities in the fetuses [2–4]. Vertical transmission of ZIKV was demonstrated by the RNA viral detection in placenta, amniotic fluid, serum and fetal brain in products with microcephaly, abortions or in autopsies of affected newborns and offspring of symptomatic or asymptomatic mothers [5, 6].

The clinical manifestations of Zika in general population and pregnant women were mild rash, conjunctivitis and low fever, although up to 80% remain asymptomatic, higher than DEN (19%) and CHIK (45%) [1, 2, 7, 8].

ZIKV is a Flavivirus with an Asian and African lineages [9, 10]. Its RNA genome (10.8 kb) encodes for a 3419-amino acid polyprotein which form a capsid (C), a membrane precursor (prM), a wrap (E) and seven non-structural proteins (NS1, NS2A, NS2B, NS3, NS4A, NS4B and NS5) [11]. ZIKV interferes with the neural development through decreased neural progenitor cells, arrest in neuronal migration and/or disruption of the maturation process of the fetus central nervous system (CNS) [12, 13]. The congenital Zika virus syndrome (CZVS) is a pattern of congenital defects associated with ZIKV infection during the pregnancy so ZIKV pathogenicity and virulence is currently studied [14–18].

The surveillance of ZIKV infection during pregnancy in endemic regions requires screening and detection of fetal morphological abnormalities [19]. An integrated intervention model for the prevention of Zika and *Aedes*-borne diseases, that includes primary health care services, gynecologists, obstetricians, pediatricians, geneticists and neurologists should be mandatory. Strategies to prevent and control the vectors and reduce the risk for diseases transmission should be strengthened, particularly for protection of women in reproductive ages [20, 21].

Here we report final the clinical manifestations observed in a cohort of pregnant women and the congenital abnormalities in fetus and newborns during a Zika transmission period (2016–2018) in South Mexico.

2. Methods

We developed a prospective study to quantify the incidence of disease and infection in a cohort of pregnant women and newborns during an epidemic period of Zika (2016–2018). One of the main objectives of the study was to know the effect of prenatal exposure to ZIKV. The cohort included pregnant women, preferably in the first trimester of pregnancy. The follow up included clinical and molecular detection of ZIKV, DEN and CHIK. Obstetric ultrasound was performed to recognize morphological abnormalities in the fetuses.

During the development of this study, information on health care was provided to pregnant women and their partners, highlighting the importance of family planning and the use of condoms as a method to prevent the transmission of ZIKV, in addition to the implementation of measures to prevent the breeding of the *Aedes aegypti* and mosquito bites at home. We also provided information about general healthy habits, family planning and prevention of sexually transmitted diseases.

2.1 Study population

After the informed consent was signed, women were interviewed, and their medical records including periconceptional and pregnancy history, were collected. The recruitment included 884 families (3993 people) from the cities of Merida, Ticul, and Progreso de Castro in the Yucatan State, South-east Mexico [16]. Merida and its metropolitan area (≈1 million inhabitants), comprises ≈50% of the Yucatan population. Progreso de Castro (37,400) and Ticul (32,000) are smaller urban areas. We enrolled consenting pregnant women from these areas from July 1, 2016 to June 2018 including pregnant women referred by physicians in primary care facilities or hospitals within the areas of our cohort study.

2.2 Clinical follow-up of pregnant women

Patient monitoring included a monthly visit for clinical assessment and sample collection (blood and urine for RTC DEN/CHIK/ZIKV), weekly follow-up by text messages, and complete access to a telephone to report any clinical signs in pregnant women, their newborns, or any family contact. Tissues as umbilical cord blood, placental, amniotic fluid and breastmilk were collected, when possible for assessment of RT-PCR RNA ZIKV (TRIOPLEX) [22]. Other biochemical tests were performed to rule out Toxoplasma, Rubella, Cytomegalovirus, Herpes, Syphilis and HIV [23]. Depending of the mother or/and fetus risks, other test such as biochemical serum test and karyotype in amniotic fluid were taken. Ultrasound scanning was performed at the first contact and every 2 months. At the first visit, a questionnaire was fill up to establish the clinical-epidemiologic profile. The follow-up ended when the pregnancy was completed by delivery or fetal loss, or the participant withdrew from the study.

2.3 Clinical follow-up of newborns

Newborn follow up included: clinical evaluation (anthropometric measurements, APGAR score and physical exam) and sample collection for RT-PCR for DEN/CHIK/ZIKV [20–22, 24]. Patients were followed up for 24 months of life for early recognition of morphological anomalies and recorded the neurological development. These evaluations included genetic, neurologic, ophthalmologic, and audiologic evaluation. Microcephaly was defined as a cranial circumference ≥2 SDs below the mean for the age and sex of the baby, following the recommendation of the World Health Organization [25–28].

2.4 Patients not initially integrated into the cohort

At the time when the cohort study was ongoing, in the Genetic Service in the center of Investigations Dr. Hideyo Noguchi/UADY received pregnant women with morphological abnormalities detected in their fetuses, or newborn patients in whom ZIKV prenatal infection was suspected. These patients were not integrated to the cohort, but a clinical follow-up was granted. Sample collections for RT-PCR for DEN/CHIK/ZIKV were offered.

3. Results

3.1 Pregnant women cohort

The study integrated 130 pregnant women with average age of 25 years. No major differences in age distribution and socioeconomic status between ZIKV-positive and ZIKV-negative mothers were observed. Of all women, 40 (30%) were in the first trimester of pregnancy upon admission to the study, 62 (48%) in the second trimester and 28 (22%) in the third trimester (**Table 1**).

Positive results in *blood/urine* for ZIKV were found in 39 pregnant women, 31% (n = 13/39) at the first trimester, 52% (n = 20/39) in the second trimester and 15% (n = 6/39) in the third trimester.

Of 130 pregnant women, 39 (30%) were RNA-ZIKV positive at the time of the recruitment and 91 were negative (70%). From these, 11 (12% of initially RNA-ZIKV negative) became positive during the surveillance.

	Total pregnant women	Positive for ZIKV in blood/urine	Negative for ZIKV in blood/urine	Trimester of pregnancy when enrolled pregnant women (130)		
	N:130	N:39	N:91	1st N:40	2nd N:62	3rd N:28
Mérida	75 (58%)	27 (69%)	47 (52%)	16 (40%)	37 (60%)	22 (79%)
Progreso	4 (3%)	0	4 (4)	0	2 (3%)	2 (7%)
Ticul	51 (39%)	12 (31%)	41 (44%)	24 (60%)	23 (37%)	4 (14%)
15–19 years	29 (22%)	8 (28%)	21 (72%)	6 (15%)	16 (26%)	7 (25%)
20–29 years	70 (54%)	22 (31%)	48 (69)	22 (55%)	34 (55%)	15 (54%)
30–39 years	30 (23%)	9 (23%)	21 (%)	12 (30%)	12 (19%)	6 (21%)
40–49 years	1 (1%)	0	1 (%)	0	0	1
Signs and symptoms		21/39 (%)				
Exanthema		21/21 (100%)				
Pruritus		11/21 (52%)				
Joint edema		7/21 (33%)				
Conjunctivitis		16/21 (76%)				
Retro-orbital pain		10/21 (55%)				
Hyperemia		5/21 (22%)				

Clinical profile in persistence in serum samples	**Total N:15**	**Symptomatic N:9**	**Asymptomatic**	**p**
Age (years)	24.7 ± 4.4	24.2 ± 3.3	23.8 ± 6	0.874
Persistence (days) (interval)	45.93 ± 24.4 (17–19)	50.11 ± 30.58 (17–97)	39.67 ± 9.89 (29–52)	0.363
Pregnancy trimester				
First	6 (40%)	3	3	
Second	8 (53%)	6	2	
Third	1 (7%)		1	

Table 1.
Summary of health, medical and laboratory data collected from pregnant women in the cohort.

Of the 28 symptomatic patients (negative or positive ZIKV), the most common symptoms were exanthema (75%), pruritus (39%) and conjunctivitis (57%). Of the 21 patients with RT-PCR ZIKV-positive, 75% were symptomatic and 25% were asymptomatic. Even so, more than half (64%) of the women had at least, more than one sign or symptom compatible with an *Aedes*-borne acute infection. Most prevalent symptoms were exanthema (100%), conjunctivitis (76%), pruritus (52%) headache (50%), retro-orbital pain (55%), arthralgia (33%), hyperemia (22%) and joint edema (6%). No hemorrhagic or systemic complications were observed in any patient (**Table 1**). Differences in the distribution of ZIKV-positive vs. ZIKV-negative women between the studied cities were not founded.

3.2 Persistence of ZIKV viral RNA in serum and urine in pregnant women

Of the 39 ZIKV-positive pregnant women, persistent RNA-ZIKV was detected in 38.5% (15/39) of the patients during 14 days after the initial symptoms or the last

PCR detection. Of these, six women were in the first trimester of gestation, eight in the second and one in the third. Within the group of symptomatic women (n = 28), nine (9/28) presented persistence of RNA-ZIKV, three in the first trimester and six

Newborn residence	**Merida N:67**		**Progreso N:2**		**Ticul N:46**		**Total births N:115**
Percentile	**Percentile <3 N (%)**		**Percentile 3–97 N (%)**		**Percentile >97 N (%)**		**Total**
	At birth	**End of the study**	**At birth**	**End of the study**	**At birth**	**End of the study**	
Birth weight percentiles	5 (4)	1 (1)	110 (96)	114 (99)	0 (0)	0 (0)	115 (100)
Birth height percentiles	3 (3)	0 (0)	112 (97)	115 (100)	0 (0)	0 (0)	115 (100)
Birth head circumference percentiles	2 (2)	1 (1)	112 (97)	114 (99)	0 (0)	0 (0)	115 (100)

Newborn evaluations				
	From mothers ZIKV negative during pregnancy N:80		**From mothers ZIKV positive during pregnancy N:35**	
	N (%)	**Alterations N (%)**	**N (%)**	**Alterations N (%)**
Newborn blood	29 (36)		27 (77)	
Newborn urine	32 (40)		14 (40)	
Pediatrics	39 (49)		30 (86)	
Ophthalmology	19 (24)		31 (89)	3 (10)
Auditory screening	51 (64)		30 (86)	2 (7)
Placenta	NA	NA	17 (49)	
Umbilical cord	NA	NA	17 (49)	
Genetics	NA	NA	35 (100)	
Metabolic screening	NA	NA	34 (97)	
Transfontanelar and abdominal ultrasound	NA	NA	22 (63)	

Age of newborns who completed the study			
Age	**Mother ZIKV –**	**Mother ZIKV +**	**Total**
1–6 months	16 (22%)	0	16 (16%)
7–12 months	25 (34%)	3 (10%)	28 (27%)
13–18 months	20 (27%)	17 (59%)	37 (36%)
19–23 months	12 (17%)	9 (31%)	21 (21%)
Total	73	29	102

Table 2.
Newborn cohort follow-up.

Patient/sex	Mother Zika symptoms (MoG[1])	WoG[2]	Neonatal head circumference (z score)	Birth weight for gestational age	Phenotype	Intracranial calcification	Zika IgM InBios newborn/mother[6]	Final diagnosis
1/Male	No	38	**Microcephaly (−3)**	Small	**Microcephaly MMC[3]**	**Yes**	−/−	CZS/neural tube defect
2/Male	**Yes (2)**	37	Normocephaly (10)	Small	IUGR[4]	NR[5]	−/−	IUGR
3/Male	No	38	**Microcephaly (−3)**	Appropriated	**Microcephaly**	**Yes**	−/−	CZS
4/Male	**Yes (2)**	37	Normocephaly (3)	Small	Asymptomatic	NR	−/−	IgM positive for toxoplasma
5/Male	No	33	Normocephaly (10)	Appropriated	**Microcephaly Arthrogryposis**	**Yes**	Positive in serum/−	CZS
6/Male	No	39	**Microcephaly (−3)**	Appropriated	**Microcephaly**	**Yes**	−/−	CZS
7/Female	**Yes (2)**	40	Normocephaly (3)	Small	**Postnatal microcephaly**	NR	−/−	CZS
8/Female	No	38	Macrocephaly (97)	Appropriated	**Macrocephaly Arthrogryposis**	Normal	−/−	Amyoplasia congenital

[1]*Month of gestation.*
[2]*Weeks of gestation.*
[3]*Myelomeningocele.*
[4]*Intrauterine growth retardation.*
[5]*NR: not reported.*
[6]*Serum and urine were taken at born in newborns and theirs mothers.*

Table 3.
Main findings of eight patients evaluated for suspected ZIKV prenatal infection.

in the second. Of these, 100% (9/9) presented rash, 55% (5/9) conjunctivitis and 33.3% (2/9) fever. Only 22.2% (2/28) reported having three symptoms, fever, rash and conjunctivitis (**Table 1**).

3.3 Newborn evaluations

All pregnancies of women in the cohort have ended the pregnancy. Two fetal losses (one in the first trimester and one in the third trimester) occurred in ZIKV-negative mothers. Of all newborns alive, 3% were preterm (two in ZIKV-negative mothers and one in a ZIKV-positive moth group). No newborns or products of conception were positive for RNA-ZIKV. Clinical evaluation of Apgar scores in the newborns did not show significant differences between positive/negative ZIKV mothers. Also, microcephaly was not founded in any newborn. One newborn of Zika-positive mother died the first days of life due to gastroschisis (**Table 2**).

During the ZIKV epidemiological period in Yucatan, 10 patients attended the medical genetics clinic in CIR Hideyo Noguchi with a reference diagnosis of microcephaly, arthrogryposis and/or ventriculomegaly. Two of them were excluded from the follow up because ZIKV prenatal symptoms were absent in the mothers and microcephaly and intracranial calcifications were discarded in the patients. Preconceptional, prenatal and perinatal backgrounds were investigated in all patients. Only one woman took folic acid 6 months before the conception and none used mosquito repellent during pregnancy, even they were living in an endemic region.

Of the newborns evaluated, clinical symptoms of Zika were reported only in two mothers in the first trimester of gestation, but only one was tested positive for RT-PCR Zika. One more woman reported symptoms of Zika 1 month before conception. During the pregnancy, intrauterine growth restriction in 4/8 (50%) and oligohydramnios in 2/8 (25%) were reported. Only one patient was reported prenatally with microcephaly, intracranial calcifications and ventriculomegaly (patient 5) (**Table 3**). Five pregnancies were ended by caesarean section and three by vaginal delivery between second semester of 2016 and the second semester of 2017.

All newborns were at term, except one. Of them, six were males and two were females. Three males had microcephaly with less than three standard deviations and one male with microcephaly less than two standard deviations. One female had macrocephaly. All babies from the three mothers with positive ZIKV symptoms during o before pregnancy were born with normocephaly, but were small for gestational age. One of these babies, a female, developed microcephaly within the first 6 months of life. Of all babies follow up, two had arthrogryposis, one with microcephaly and one with macrocephaly. Both of them were child from non-symptomatic mothers. Only five patients were evaluated with axial computerized tomography with positive intracranial calcifications founded in four. All of them were from asymptomatic mothers.

All patients and their mothers were tested for RT-PCR for ZIKV/DEN/CHIK in serum and urine. TORCH was also performed. RNA-ZIKV was obtained only in serum of one male with microcephaly, arthrogryposis and intracranial calcifications. This male was from an asymptomatic mother. Antibodies IgM of toxoplasma were detected in one asymptomatic male whom has clinical symptoms of Zika during first trimester of pregnancy.

4. Discussion

The WHO declared the ZIKV outbreak in South America and the associated increase in neurological disorders and neonatal malformations a "*public health emergency of international concern*" [2], and the CDC issued the ZIKV epidemiological alert, recommendations of high-risk Mexican territories was recognized by the National Health Service. Even so, the recognition of the ZIKV infection symptoms by patients and health workers, were underestimated [29]. In Mexico, first patients with ZIKV infection were documented early in 2016 even so, captured mosquitoes in early 2015 were recognized with ZIKV infection [30].

After the observed relationship between prenatal Zika infection and the risk of congenital defects in Brazil and Colombia, we realized a cohort with detailed evaluation of pregnant women searching ZIKV infection and congenital abnormalities [1, 31, 32].

The women in this study with the highest proportion of symptoms with ZIKV were those from 20 to 29 years, different from other studies that have reported the highest symptomatic disease ratio among women >30 years of age [33, 34]. In our studies this can be explained because the highest incidence of pregnancies in women was aged 20–29 years [1]. In clinically affected women, univariate analyzes showed that the most sensitive clinical sign was the exanthema, but it was also the least specific. The triad, conjunctival hyperemia, joint edema and exanthema had the highest level of specificity [35].

In pregnant women with exanthema without fever or other symptoms should to suspect ZIKV infection. In this study, ZIKV/DEN/CHIK co-infection was not identified neither [36].

The persistence of RNA viral in pregnant women has been described previously, reported a patient positive for RNA-ZIKV until 10 weeks after the onset of symptoms. In this study, the maximum viremia persistence was 97 days, but a quarter of positive mothers had viremia for more than 8 weeks [37]. From all RNA ZIKV-positive mothers, only 50% of the symptomatic group had persistence of ZIKV for more than 8 weeks. Other series reported longer RNA ZIKV viremia in symptomatic women than asymptomatic and other study obtained similar results in serum, in a range of 14–63 days; although in this study, we detected two pregnant women who had viremia older than 90 days [33, 34]. A study reported viral persistence in five pregnant women, of which 80% were symptomatic and only one case was asymptomatic. In this study, a higher percentage of asymptomatic viral persistence cases were found with 40%. In the symptomatic group, the average number of days of persistence after the onset of symptoms was greater than that reported, no relationship was observed between viral persistence and the presence of abnormalities in pregnancy products [38, 39].

The confirmatory tests which provide evidence for prenatal infection by ZIKV were conducted based on tests in the mother and the newborn were made with viral RNA isolated from biological fluids and placental tissues performed with the Trioplex kit of the CDC. The ZIKV genome was detected in cerebrospinal fluid, cardiac fluid, chorionic villi, fetal face of the placenta, serum and urine [26]. Vertical transmission studying the placental and fetus tissue also failed been demonstrated [40, 41].

Clinical variability in patients in whom ZIKV infection were prenatally suspected was described previously, in this cohort, congenital abnormalities associated to ZIKV were not observed in fetus, stillborn or newborns [1, 17]. Only one patient with gastroschisis was detected but the prenatal ZIKV infection in her mother was after detection of this abnormality.

Congenital Zika syndrome (CSZ) was observed in the patients evaluated from the Genetics Service out of the initial cohort. In them, Zika symptoms in mothers, microcephaly, arthrogryposis and intracranial calcifications were observed as in other reports [1, 17, 18]. Establishing the final diagnosis of ZIKV prenatal infection was difficult especially in asymptomatic mothers or in mild affected babies [31].

In two patients, the final diagnosis was toxoplasma and congenital amyoplasia. Asymptomatic or mild symptomatic women would be a seriously limitation from early ZIKV infection. To define diagnostic of prenatal ZIKV is important: (1) to establish the follow up of the affected patient, (2) to limit the tests related to others genetic diseases that share symptoms with CSZ and (3) to establish the specific risk of recurrences of congenital abnormalities in subsequent pregnancies in the mother.

5. Conclusions

In this study, symptomatic or asymptomatic pregnant women with a high prevalence for ZIKV are reported, however there was no positive newborn or with malformations associated with ZIKV, despite the genetic consultation, the presence of CSZ, laboratory-confirmed if present so doctors should maintain a realistic perspective of the impact of ZIKV on pregnancy. And despite the uncertainties, future mothers should receive adequate, systematic advice and the best planned obstetric surveillance, always considering the gestational moment of maternal ZIKV infection and accept that there is gestational risk for different elements of the CZS phenotype in risk areas ZIKV transmission.

Acknowledgements

This research and publication was made possible through support provided by and the Canadian Institutes of Health Research (CIHR) and IDRC (preventing Zika disease with novel vector control approaches Project 108412) and the Office of Infectious Disease, Bureau for Global Health, US Agency for International Development, under the terms of an Interagency Agreement with CDC. The opinions expressed herein are those of the author(s) and do not necessarily reflect the views of the US Agency for International Development. The recipient of this support was the Yucatan Autonomous University and its affiliated Regional Research Center "Hideyo Noguchi."

Author details

Norma Pavía-Ruz[1], Silvina Noemí Contreras-Capetillo[1], Yamila Romer[2], Nina Valadez Gonzalez[1], Hector Gómez-Dantés[3], Gonzalo Vázquez-Prokopec[2] and Pablo Manrique-Saide[1*]

1 Autonomous University de Yucatan, Merida, Yucatan, Mexico

2 Emory University, Atlanta, GA, USA

3 Public Health Institute of Mexico, Cuernavaca, Morelos, México

*Address all correspondence to: msaide@correo.uady.mx; pablo_manrique2000@hotmail.com

References

[1] Brasil P, Pereira JP, Raja Gabaglia C, Damasceno L, Wakimoto M, Ribeiro Nogueira RM, et al. Zika virus infection in pregnant women in Rio de Janeiro—Preliminary report. The New England Journal of Medicine. 2016. DOI: 10.1056/NEJMoa1602412

[2] Reynolds MR, Jones AM, Petersen EE, Lee EH, Rice ME, Bingham A, et al. Vital signs: Update on Zika virus-associated birth defects and evaluation of all U.S. infants with congenital Zika virus exposure—U.S. Zika pregnancy. MMWR. 2017;**66**:1-9

[3] Venancio FA, Quilião Bernal ME, Vieira Ramos MCB, Rocha Chaves N, Hendges MV, Marques Rodrigues de Souza M, et al. Congenital Zika syndrome in a Brazil-Paraguay-Bolivia border region: Clinical features of cases diagnosed between 2015 and 2018. PLoS ONE. 2019;**14**(10):e0223408. DOI: 10.1371/journal.pone.0223408

[4] World Health Organization. Zika situation report. [Accessed: 5 February 2016]. Available at: http://www.who.int/emergencies/zika-virus/situation-report/5-february-2016/en/

[5] Besnard M, Lastère S, Teissier A, Cao-Lormeau VM, Musso D. Evidence of perinatal transmission of Zika virus, French Polynesia, December 2013 and February 2014. Euro Surveillance. 2014;**19**:1-4

[6] Calvet G, Aguiar RS, Melo ASO, Sampaio SA, de Filippis I, Fabri A, et al. Detection and sequencing of Zika virus from amniotic fluid of fetuses with microcephaly in Brazil: A case study. The Lancet Infectious Diseases. 2016;**16**:653-660

[7] Rojas DP, Barrera-Fuentes GA, Pavia-Ruz N, Salgado-Rodriguez M, Che-Mendoza A, Manrique-Saide P, et al. Epidemiology of dengue and other arboviruses in a cohort of school children and their families in Yucatan, Mexico: Baseline and first year follow-up. PLoS Neglected Tropical Diseases. 2018;**12**(11):e0006847. DOI: 10.1371/journal.pntd.0006847

[8] Pavía-Ruz N, Villanueva S, Granja P, Balam-May A, Longini IM, Halloran ME, et al. Seroprevalence of dengue antibodies in three urban settings in Yucatan, Mexico. American Journal of Tropical Medicine and Hygiene. 2018;**98**:1202-1208. DOI: 10.4269/ajtmh.17-0382

[9] Haddow AD, Schuh AJ, Yasuda CY, Kasper MR, Heang V, Huy R, et al. Genetic characterization of Zika virus strains: Geographic expansion of the Asian lineage. PLoS Neglected Tropical Diseases. 2012;**6**(2):e1477. DOI: 10.1371/journal.pntd.0001477

[10] Rinkenberger N, Schoggins JW. Comparative analysis of viral entry for Asian and African lineages of Zika virus. Virology. 2019;**533**:59-67

[11] Xing H, Xu S, Jia F, et al. Zika NS2B is a crucial factor recruiting NS3 to the ER and activating its protease activity. Virus Research. 2020;**275**:197793. DOI: 10.1016/j.virusres.2019.197793

[12] Annamalai AS, Pattnaik A, Sahoo BR, Muthukrishnan E, Natarajan SK, Steffen D, et al. Zika virus encoding nonglycosylated envelope protein is attenuated and defective in neuroinvasion. Journal of Virology. 2017;**91**:e01348-e01317. DOI: 10.1128/JVI.01348-17

[13] Leda AR, Bertrand L, Andras IE, El-Hage N, Nair M, Toborek M. Selective disruption of the blood-brain barrier by Zika virus. Frontiers in Microbiology. 2019;**10**:2158. DOI: 10.3389/fmicb.2019.02158

[14] Beys-da-Silva WO, Rosa RL, Santi L, Berger M, Park SK, Campos AR, et al. Zika virus infection of human mesenchymal stem cells promotes differential expression of proteins linked to several neurological diseases. Molecular Neurobiology. 2019;**56**(7):4708-4717. DOI: 10.1007/s12035-018-1417-x

[15] Shao Q, Herrlinger S, Yang S-L, Lai F, Moore JM, Brindley MA, et al. Zika virus infection disrupts neurovascular development and results in postnatal microcephaly with brain damage. Development. 2016;**143**(22):4127-4136. DOI: 10.1242/dev.143768

[16] Acosta-Reyes J, Navarro E, Herrera MJ, Goenaga E, Ospina ML, Parra E, et al. Severe neurologic disorders in 2 fetuses with Zika virus infection, Colombia. Emerging Infectious Diseases. 2017;**23**:982-984. DOI: 10.3201/eid2306.161702

[17] Del Campo M, Feitosa IM, Ribeiro EM, Horovitz DD, Pessoa AL, França GV, et al. The phenotypic spectrum of congenital Zika syndrome. American Journal of Medical Genetics. 2017;**173**:841-857. DOI: 10.1002/ajmg.a.38170

[18] Moore CA, Stables JE, Dobyns WB, Pessoa A, Ventura CV, Fonseca EB, et al. Characterizing the pattern of anomalies in congenital Zika syndrome for pediatric clinicians. JAMA Pediatrics. 2017;**171**(3):288-2995. DOI: 10.1001/jamapediatrics.2016.3982

[19] Lebov JF, Arias JF, Balmaseda A, Britt W, Cordero JF, Galvão LA, et al. International prospective observational cohort study of Zika in infants and pregnancy (ZIP study): Study protocol. BMC Pregnancy and Childbirth. 2019;**19**:282. DOI: 10.1186/s12884-019-2430-4

[20] Romer Y, Valadez-Gonzalez N, Contreras-Capetillo S, Manrique-Saide P, Vazquez-Prokopec G, Pavia-Ruz N. Zika virus infection in pregnant women, Yucatan, Mexico. Emerging Infectious Diseases. 2019;**25**:1452-1460

[21] Pavía-Ruz N, Contreras-Capetillo S, Valadez-González N, Villegas-Chim J, Carcaño-Castillo R, Valencia-Pacheco G, et al. Current Topics in Zika: An Integrated Intervention Model for the Prevention of Zika and Other Aedes-Borne Diseases in Women and Their Families in Mexico. IntechOpen; 2018. ISBN: 978953.51-0317-2

[22] Colombo TE, Versiani AF, Dutra KR, et al. Performance of CDC Trioplex qPCR during a dengue outbreak in Brazil. Journal of Clinical Virology. 2019;**121**:104208. DOI: 10.1016/j.jcv.2019.104208

[23] Oduyabo T, Petersen EE, Rasmussen AA, Mead PS, Meaney-Delman D, Renquist CM, et al. Update: Interim guidelines for health care providers caring for pregnant women and women of reproductive age with possible Zika virus exposure—United States, 2016. MMWR. 2016;**65**(5):122-127

[24] Casey BM, McIntire DD, Leveno KJ. The continuing value of the Apgar score for the assessment of newborn infants. The New England Journal of Medicine. 2001;**344**:46771. DOI: 10.1056/NEJM200102153440701

[25] Lanciotti RS, Kosoy OL, Laven JJ, Velez JO, Lambert AJ, Johnson AJ, et al. Genetic and serologic properties of Zika virus associated with an epidemic, Yap State, Micronesia, 2007. Emerging Infectious Diseases. 2008;**4**:1232-1239. DOI: 10.3201/eid1408.080287

[26] Rabe IB, Staples JE, Villanueva J, Hummel KB, Johnson JA, Rose L, et al. Interim guidance for interpretation of Zika virus antibody test results. MMWR. Morbidity and Mortality

Weekly Report. 2016;**65**:543-546. DOI: 10155_85/mmwr.mm6521e1

[27] Bhatnagar J, Rabeneck DB, Martines RB, Reagan-Steiner S, Ermias Y, Estetter B, et al. Zika virus RNA replication and persistence in brain and placental tissue. Emerging Infectious Diseases. 2017;**23**:405-414. DOI: 10.3201/eid2303.161499

[28] Centers for Disease Control and Prevention. Revised diagnostic testing for Zika, Chikungunya, and dengue viruses in US public health laboratories. [Cited: 31 August 2017]. Available from: https://www.cdc.gov/zika/transmission/index.htlm

[29] Flemming-Dutra KE, Nelson JM, Fischer M, Staples E, Karwowski MP, Mead O, et al. Update: Interim guidelines for health care provider caring for infants and children with possible Zika virus infection-United States, February 2016. MMWR. 2016;**65**:1-6

[30] Díaz-Quiñonez JA, López-Martínez I, Torres-Longoria B, Vázquez-Pichardo M, Cruz-Ramírez E, Ramírez-González JE, et al. Evidence of the presence of the Zika virus in Mexico since early 2015. Virus Genes. 2016;**52**(6):855-857

[31] Contreras-Capetillo SN, Valadéz-González N, Manrique-Saide P, Carcaño-Castillo RE, Pacheco-Tugores F, Barrera-Pérez HAM, et al. Birth defects associated with congenital Zika virus infection in Mexico. Clinical Pediatrics. 2017;**10**:1-10

[32] Alvarado-Socarras JL, Ocampo-González M, Vargas-Soler JA, Rodríguez-Morales AJ, Franco-Paredes C. Congenital and neonatal chikungunya in Colombia. Journal of the Pediatric Infectious Diseases Society. 2016;**5**:e17-e20

[33] Duffy MR, Chen T-H, Hancock WT, Powers AM, Kool JL, Lanciotti RS, et al. Zika virus outbreak on Yap Island, Federated States of Micronesia. The New England Journal of Medicine. 2009;**360**:253643. DOI: 10.1056/NEJMoa0805715

[34] Flamand C, Fritzell C, Matheus S, Dueymes M, Carles G, Favre A, et al. The proportion of asymptomatic infections and spectrum of disease among pregnant women infected by Zika virus: Systematic monitoring in French Guiana, 2016. Euro Surveillance. 2017;**22**. DOI: 10.2807/1560-7917.ES.2017.22.44.17-00102

[35] Nicastri E, Pisapia R, Corpolongo A, Fusco FM, Cicalini S, Scognamiglio P, et al. Three cases of zika virus imported in Italy: Need for a clinical awareness and evidence-based knowledge. BMC Infectious Diseases. 2016;**16**:66960

[36] Vogels CBF, Rückert C, Cavany SM, Perkins TA, Ebel G, Grubaugh ND. Arbovirus coinfection and co-transmission: A neglected public health concern? PLoS Biology. 2019;**17**(1):e3000130. DOI: 10.1371/journal.pbio.3000130

[37] Salehuddin AR, Haslan H, Mamikutty N, Zaidun NH, Azmi MF, Senin MM, et al. Zika virus infection and its emerging trends in Southeast Asia. Asian Pacific Journal of Tropical Medicine. 2017;**10**(3):211-219

[38] Driggers RW, Korhonen EM, Kuivanen S, Jääskeläinen AJ, Smura T, Rosenberg A, et al. Zika virus infection with prolonged maternal viremia and fetal brain abnormalities. The New England Journal of Medicine. 2016. DOI: 10.1056/NEJMoa1601824

[39] Meaney-Delman D, Oduyebo T, Polen KN, White JL, Bingham AM, Slavinski SA, et al. Prolonged detection of Zika virus RNA in pregnant women. Obstetrics and Gynecology. 2016;**128**(4):724-730

[40] Paz-Bailey G, Rosenberg ES, Doyle K, Munoz-Jordan J, Santiago GA, Klein L, et al. Persistence of Zika virus in body fluids—Final report. The New England Journal of Medicine. 2017;**379**(13):1234-1243. DOI: 10.1056/NEJMoa1613108

[41] Besnard M, Lastére S, Teissier A, Cao-Lourmeau VM, Musso D. Evidence of perinatal transmission of Zika virus, French Polynesia, December 2013 and February 2014. Euro Surveillance. 2014;**19**(13):1-4

Chapter 5

The Eye and the Zika Virus

Dayron Fernando Martínez-Pulgarín,
Carlos Miguel Córdoba-Ortega
and Fabio Daniel Padilla-Pantoja

Abstract

Ocular involvement in Zika virus (ZIKV) infection can be present both in adults and infants as acquired and congenital diseases respectively. Through experimental studies, there has been clarified important mechanisms of ocular pathogenesis that allow the establishment of potential objectives for antiviral drugs development. The spread of the virus at the ocular level could be hematogenous or axonal, however the hematogenous route through the choroid is suggested as the most important initial mechanism for infection. Ocular manifestations vary according to the age of presentation, being mild and self-limited in adults and potentially devastating in children, related to congenital Zika syndrome (CZS). Ocular diagnosis is made based in clinical features and contact/travel history to countries of epidemiological importance; fundoscopy, optical coherence tomography, fluoresceinic/green indocianine angiography, cultures, serological and molecular tests are useful diagnostic tools. Ocular management is focused according to the clinical context of each patient. Prevention is carried out in a comprehensive manner and further research is directed to vaccine development and specific antiviral treatment. Proper attention requires a multidisciplinary team in order to reach complete visual evaluation and early rehabilitation.

Keywords: Zika virus, congenital Zika syndrome, uveitis, optic nerve hypoplasia, conjunctivitis

1. Introduction

Zika virus (ZIKV) is a mosquito-borne viral disease caused by a flavivirus from the Flaviviridae family and transmitted by species belonging mainly to genus Aedes, discovered in 1947 in Uganda in infected rhesus monkeys [1, 2] with the first human cases reported in Africa and Asia [3]. Latin America and the Caribbean started to be affected with outbreaks, the first one reported in 2015 in Brazil [4]. Systemic symptoms include fever, maculo-papular rash, headache, arthralgia and conjunctivitis [2, 5].

Ocular involvement of ZIKV is not an uncommon manifestation in a patient with Zika virus infection. There are two main situations in which ocular pathology can occur: The first one is the manifestation of the virus in an adult patient, including the non-purulent conjunctivitis and more rarely ocular inflammation, especially in the anterior segment [6, 7]. Non-purulent conjunctivitis occurs between 55 and 63% of patients, as reported in outbreaks from Yap Islands and French Polineise, however according to other studies, conjunctivitis only occurs between 10 and 25% of patients infected with ZIKV [8–10].

The second way implies ocular abnormalities of congenital etiology, that belongs to the congenital Zika syndrome (CZS) [11]. The most prevalent congenital disorder is brain calcifications (42.6; 95%CI, 30.8–54.4), meanwhile the prevalence of ocular disorders was less frequent (4.2; 95% CI, 1.0–7.5) [10]. The overall presentation rate of ocular manifestations in infants with CZS is 21.4–55% [11, 12]. Infection due to ZIKV in the first trimester of pregnancy can trigger the presentation of CZS in 1–13% of the cases with ocular manifestations in patients present up to 70% of cases [13].

First report in literature about ocular manifestation in CZS was published in 2016 with three cases of children with mothers exposed to the virus during gestational age, leading to macular chorioretinal atrophy in all cases [14]. A second report of ocular anomalies related to CZS was done in a 10 case-series, informing horizontal nystagmus in 10% of cases, exophoria in 40% of cases, esophoria in 20% of cases, macular alterations like gross pigment mottling and/or chorioretinal atrophy and optic nerve anomalies like hypoplasia with double-ring sign, pallor, and/or increased cup-to-disk ratio in 75 and 45% of evaluated eyes respectively [15]. An interesting fact about these ocular anomalies is that it is not required the presence of microcephaly to get an ocular involvement, like was reported by Ventura et al. in an infant with cerebral calcifications and an unilateral chorioretinal scar in macular region [16] .

In the same year, it was reported a case series including 29 patients with microcephaly due to CZS, in which 36.5% had some degree of ocular involvement: Lens subluxation, bilateral iris coloboma, optic nerve abnormalities and chorioretinal atrophy in 5.9, 11.8, 47.1 and 64.7% of cases respectively [17]. Afterwards, in 2017, in a bigger sample (70 children with microcephaly),36% were positive to ophthalmological findings like macular and optic nerve anomalies (26% of ocular cases), strabismus/nystagmus (10% of ocular cases) and suboptimal visual acuity (100% of ocular cases) [18]. Zin et al. reported a cohort of 112 children with 21.4% of cases with positive ocular findings: 79.2% of cases with optic nerve abnormalities, 58.3% with retinal involvement, 25% with nystagmus, 4.2% with microphthalmia [19].

In Colombia and near countries like Venezuela, exists studies reporting ocular findings [20], like a study with 43 microcephalic children, of which 12% presented optic nerve hypoplasia, 63% macular pigment mottling, 7% lacunar maculopathy and 12% developed congenital glaucoma [21]. Alvarado-Socarras et al. reported a case series of children born from women infected with ZIKV, where two children had intraretinal hemorrhages, hyper/hypopigmented lesions. The increased risk for ocular ZIKV in these cases where derived from the presence of microcephaly and the infection during pregnancy [22].

In an attempt to assess the risk factors associated to ocular manifestations, Ventura et al. conducted a cross-sectional study including 40 microcephalic children, 60% of them with ZIKV positive infection. There was a statistically significant relationship of ocular manifestations to children with smaller cephalic diameter at birth (95%CI, −2.56 to −0.51; P = 0.004) and infants whose mothers reported symptoms during the first trimester (95%CI, 0.02–0.67; P = 0.04) [23]. It is relevant to mention that not only ocular structural changes are manifest in children with CZS, but also functional abnormalities like ocular motor disorders, visual fields defects (45.1% of cases), low contrast sensitivity (81.3% of cases), hypoaccomodation and refractive errors. Prevalence rate of severe visual impairment without structural changes is present in 84.6% of cases, related to cortical/cerebral involvement [24]. According to Baran et al., visual acuity losses occur in children with gestational infection, with a slowing of visual development even in the absence of microcephaly [25].

It is not necessary the presence of microcephaly in children or ZIKV systemic symptoms in pregnant women to manifest ocular abnormalities. Ocular involvement caused by Zika virus should be included in differential diagnosis, especially in endemic areas, of any patient presenting ocular manifestations and a history of fever. This chapter describes the most important aspects of the ocular compromise caused by ZIKV, items that the clinicians should consider when approaching a patient with a suspected ocular involvement by the mentioned virus.

2. Ocular pathogenesis

ZIKV, similar to other flaviviruses, has an icosahedral envelope with positive single-stranded RNA as a genetic material that encodes a polyprotein processed by viral and cellular proteases into three structural proteins: capsid proteins, membrane and envelope that form the viral particle and mediate the binding of the virus, allowing entry and encapsidation. Seven non-structural proteins (NS) (NS1, NS2A, NS2B, NS3, NS4A, NS4B and NS5), play a role for polyproteins processing and the induction of an innate antiviral response in the host. The main surface glycoprotein involved in the binding of the host cell and the fusion of the viral membrane is the envelope protein, which allows the fixation and fusion of the viral particle to the host cell and is a useful tool in the diagnosis [26]. Viral reproduction is achieved through non-structural proteins (NS1–NS5), which serve as self-dividing peptidases, together with viral RNA-dependent RNA polymerase [27].

Through the endocytosis process, the virion enters the cytoplasm of the cells [28]. Non-structural proteins bind to the endoplasmic reticulum, where viral replication of RNA is performed using cell structure and dynamics and released by cellular apoptosis. Subsequently, it takes the viral phase that occurs between 3 and 5 days after the first symptoms, then hematogenous spread to organs and tissues occurs. It is believed that the virus could have neuronal (pantropic) and other organ tropism, because viral RNA has been found in the brain, as well as in the liver, kidney, heart and spleen [29]. There are also other forms of transmission called non-vector, such as vertical transmission [30, 31], sexual transmission and blood transfusion [32, 33].

The pathophysiology of the ocular findings is not known in detail so far. It has been studied in animal models and deceased fetuses that have tried to demonstrate the great retinal compromise that includes macular abnormalities such as pigment spots and chorioretinal atrophy, loss of retinal pigment epithelium, perivascular choroidal inflammatory infiltrate and optic nerve abnormalities such as hypoplasia, paleness and increased cup-disc ratio. Other publications describe additional findings, such as iris coloboma, lens subluxation, cataracts, glaucoma, and microphthalmia [15, 34, 35]. At the ocular level, Zika virus infection can affect any part of the uveal tract (iris, ciliary body, retina and choroid), since most clinical cases have defects in the posterior segment [14, 15]. The hematoretinal barrier formed by vascular endothelial cells of the inner retina and external RPE (Retinal Pigment Epithelium) cells constitutes the first protective barrier that is responsible to control the entry of innate immune cells and pathogens into the posterior eye segment [36, 37]. The type I interferon (IFN) response is an important defense mechanism against most flaviviruses. A129 mice, which are deficient in IFN α and β receptors, have been commonly used as an animal model to study ZIKV infection [38, 39].

By detection of RNA nucleic acids in animal models, it has been suggested that the ocular infection can spread hematogenously to the brain and the eye simultaneously, although it is not possible to rule out the transfer through the optic nerve, in which there has been shown that houses the higher concentration of viral antigen. Therefore, the spread of the virus at the ocular level could be hematogenous or axonal, as studies show, however the viral peak during viremia suggests the hematogenous route through the choroid choroid as a more important initial mechanism. After day 3, the progressive increase in viral RNA levels in the eye is markedly different from that of peripheral blood [40]. In a hypothetical study using human target cells, it was shown that the pathophysiology of ocular ZIKV begins when it spreads throughout the retinal bed through the retinal arteries affecting the endothelial cells and the retinal pericytes of the internal hematoretinal barrier and then compromises the choroid to infect the external hematoretinal barrier by compromising the RPE cells and allowing the amplification and spread of the virus in the retinal bed. It was found that retinal endothelial cells are highly permissive for ZIKV and showed important cytopathic effects. It was shown that Müller cells are not permissive for ZIKV infection and photoreceptor cells appear to be even less so. The highest levels of ZIKV transcription were observed in retinal pericytes [41].

It has been documented that the entry and binding of several viruses at the cellular level is facilitated by the TAM (tyrosine kinase) receptors as well as the TLR [36] (toll like receptor) that play an important role in the organization of the innate responses of the retina in the microbial infection. Among them, AXL (TAM type receptor) was identified as the main receptor involved and together with the TLR3 (toll like receptor) that is involved in the viral infection, they allow the binding of the virus and its respective anchorage to the cellular guest machinery. These findings suggest that ZIKV can use AXL as an input receptor to gain access to hematoretinal barrier cells and therefore cause retinal pathology. Host cells employ intracellular pathogen recognition receptors, such as TLR and RIG-I-like receptors, for the recognition and initiation of innate immune responses, in particular with the generation of the interferon pathway (IFN type I). ISG15 induced by type I IFN is generally considered an antiviral gene that plays a protective role in the retina against ZIKV infection. Although, ISG15 has been shown to influence viral replication both positively and negatively. The expression of several IFN-induced antiviral genes has also been demonstrated, including OAS2 and MX1 [40–42].

In animal models it has been seen that by day 9 of the infection process, there is activation of local glial cells and the start of cell recruitment given a subtle increase in the gene expression of MHC, B2m and STAT1. In addition, there is an increase in TNFα, granzyme, perforin and IFNγ without evidence of CD3 or CD8 T markers, suggesting that possibly NK cells reach the eye in the early stages of the disease [40, 42]. A few days later (days 12–16), when mice develop clinical signs of encephalitis, chemokine expression in the eyes peaks. The analysis of the profile of cytokines and adhesion molecules reveals a marginal increase in the levels of β2-m, GMCSF and MCP1 and a moderate increase in the expression of ICAM-1, IL-6 and VCAM-1; and higher levels of RANTES expression (Regulators after activation, normal T cells expressed and presumably secreted) are evidenced in ZIKV infected cells. This elevation recruits inflammatory cells in the retinal microenvironment and produces chronicity [41]. Recent studies in mouse models suggest that ZIKV is located in the iridocorneal angle and in the trabecular meshwork where through the already mentioned mechanisms, they induce cell death at the level of the trabecular meshwork, leading to induction of inflammatory response that causes trabeculitis and could be one of the potential mechanisms for the IOP increase and glaucomatous pathology [43]. Furthermore, once the infection is located at the ocular level, panuveitis can be generated in the presence of ZIKV in the layers of the cornea, choroid, bipolar and ganglion cells of the retina and optic nerve and therefore the viral RNA can be secreted from tear glands or detached from the cornea to the tears [44].

Several studies have been conducted in animal models to try to address the pathophysiological mechanism involved in the development of eye disorders. Van den Pol et al. studied an animal model in infected newborn mice, which exhibit a brain development process similar to the human brain fetus in the second trimester. They mainly analyzed the brain and the visual pathway, identifying the damage caused by ZIKV in the entire visual system, including the retina, the optic chiasma, the suprachiasmatic nucleus, the lateral geniculate nucleus and/or the superior colliculus. The theory postulated that ZIKV can be transported axonally, which improves the spread of the virus within the brain, with a fundamental role of glial cells to understand the mechanism behind neurological and ocular findings [45].

Singh et al. also conducted an animal model study that only analyzed the pathophysiology of retinal findings demonstrating that retinal cells, including those of the RPE, are permissible for ZIKV replication and express receptors for them. In addition, they are susceptible to ZIKV-induced cell death, leading to retinal lesions because of the virus ability to break the integrity of the hematoretinal barrier. They suggested that ISG15 (Interferon-stimulated gene 15) and its antiviral activity, plays a role in the innate defense of the retina against ZIKV infection [46].

In a subsequent study with a murine model, Zhao et al. showed that ZIKV can infect the retina in immunodeficient and immunocompetent mice and affect multiple retinal layers. ZIKV preferentially infects RPE and Müller cells, which are key support cells for neuronal survival, function and repair of retinal lesions. Müller cell ablation causes neurological and vascular pathological effects that resemble the ocular characteristics of congenital eye disease due to ZIKV. Müller cells show a decreased neurotrophic function with a post-infection up-regulation of cytokines

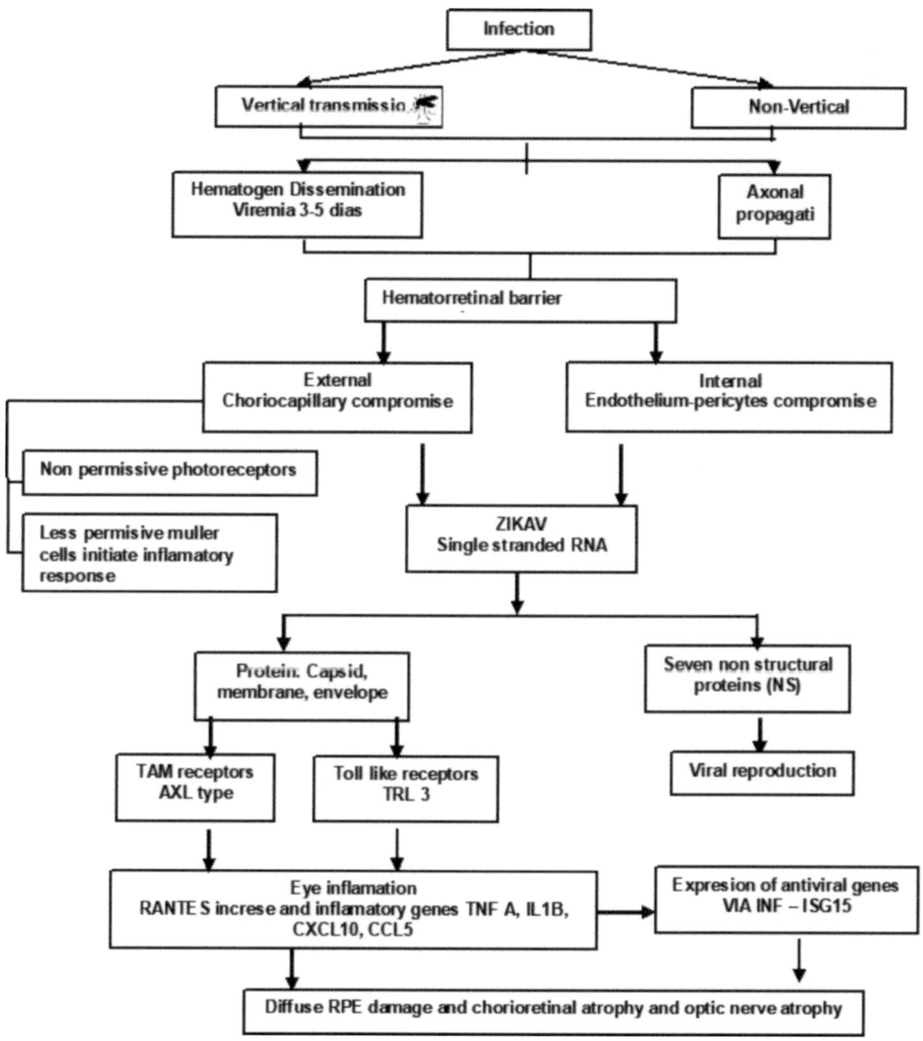

Figure 1.
Pathogenic infection process by ZIKV to the retinal pigment epithelium.

levels [47]. In a more recent study, Aleman et al. [48]. provided the first evidence in-vivo in humans that shows central retinal degeneration with severe loss of ganglion cells and a borderline thinning of nerve fibers, as well as a less prominent loss of photoreceptors. The findings provide the first evidence to date, in humans, that ganglion cells -and perhaps surrounding glia cells- are the primary cellular targets in the retina of patients with ZIKV infection, which is consistent with the murine disease model that suggest a depletion of this neuronal population in the uterus as a result of the infection [44]. **Figure 1**, resumes some of the pathogenic theories involving the ZIKV and its infection to some of the retinal cells.

3. Ophthalmologic manifestations

3.1 Ocular findings in infants with congenital Zika virus infection

The most important findings of ophthalmologic abnormalities associated with Zika virus infection are reported in infants with microcephaly due to Zika congenital infection, leading to a broad spectrum of ophthalmological manifestations. It is proposed that the ocular findings could be a result of the direct effect of Zika virus itself and not only a consequence of microcephaly, because of the known deleterious effects of the virus on the central nervous system [14, 49–51]. The increased neurotropism of the virus explains why the retina and optic nerve are the main structures affected in infants with congenital Zika virus syndrome. It has been proposed that the typical optic nerve hypoplasia is more related to microcephaly, and the retinal anomalies specially found in the neurosensory retina are associated to an inflammatory reaction due to the virus toxin. The majority of findings are bilateral [23, 52]. There is no report of uveitis in congenital cases [53].

Zika exposure without infection during gestation does not seem to affect ocular status, visual acuity or visual development. When the Zika virus is vertically transmitted to the fetus and the subsequent infection is confirmed, the infant may show ophthalmologic and visual function damage. There has been described retinal abnormalities in children with microcephaly attributed to Zika virus infection during pregnancy, found in 60–85% of the affected patients with ocular findings, including optic nerve abnormalities and macular alterations [23, 51]. It is hypothesized that the most sever ophthalmic manifestations occur when the infection takes place in the first or second trimester of pregnancy, because of the Zika's tropism related to the neural precursors, which are available in the early phases of cerebral differentiation [10, 23, 54, 55]. It has been found that retinal findings are more prevalent when the infection takes place in the first trimester and the related viral load may be relevant to the final process that results affecting the macula. In the other hand, the optic nerve could be affected in all trimesters [5].

3.1.1 Optic nerve findings and macular abnormalities

Optic nerve hypoplasia is one of the most important findings in infants with congenital Zika virus infection [51]. This condition can be identified with the double ring sign as a manifestation of a small and undeveloped optic nerve [23, 52, 56, 57] (**Figure 1**). Other typical signs of insult to the optic nerve include pallor and increased cup-to-disk ratio [13, 15, 56, 57] (**Figure 2**). The most frequent macular findings associated with congenital Zika virus infection include gross pigment mottling, foveal reflex loss and chorioretinal atrophy, which differs from toxoplasmosis scars because of the absence of intraocular inflammatory signs and the presentation of a typical dark pigmentation rim around the atrophic area [15, 18, 58].

The circumscribed macular atrophy observed in the affected children seems to be pathognomonic to congenital Zika syndrome [5, 6, 50]. The macular atrophy caused by Zika virus infection is mostly associated with involvement of the outer retinal layers and choriocapillaris (**Figure 3**). Inner retinal vascular abnormalities could also be present and associated with post-viral neurological sequelae of Zika virus infection, in addition to the well-known outer retinal effects of the infectious disease [59].

3.1.2 Anterior segment findings

Anterior ocular findings related to Zika virus infection include iris coloboma, cataracts, lens subluxation, intraocular calcifications and microphthalmia even in the absence of microcephaly [34, 60]. However, it is known that the incidence of structural eye alterations, visual acuity loss and fundus abnormalities are significantly higher when the infected child exhibits concomitant microcephaly [14, 25].

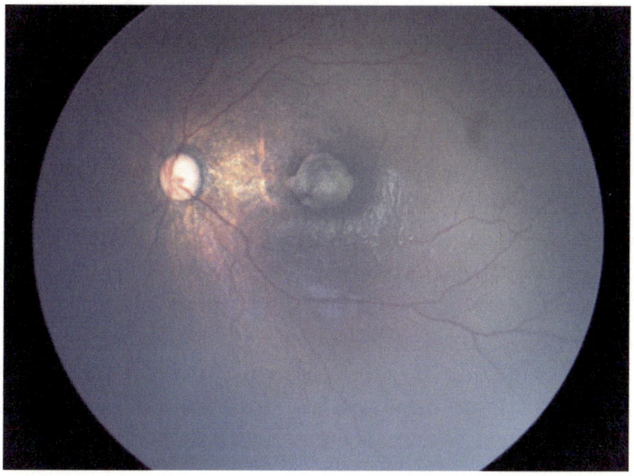

Figure 2.
Optic disc hypoplasia with double-ring sign associated with hyperpigmented mottling and one sharply demarcated chorioretinal atrophy on the macula. Image courtesy from Camila Ventura, MD, PhD. Altino Ventura foundation (FAV) - HOPE eye hospital. reproduced with permission.

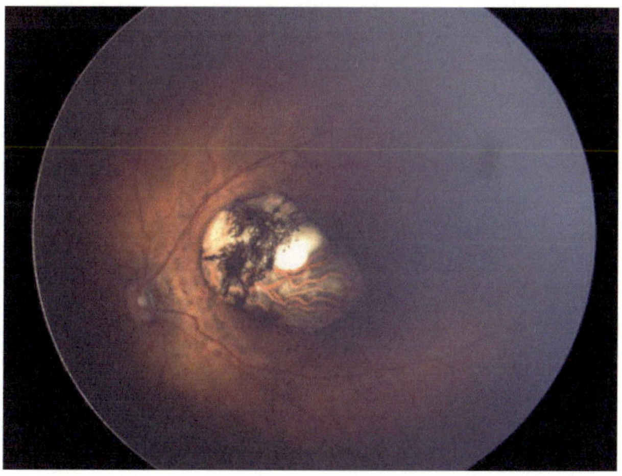

Figure 3.
Macular chorioretinal atrophy, hyperpigmented mottling, vascular attenuation and optic disc hypoplasia. Image courtesy of Camila Ventura, MD, PhD. Altino Ventura foundation (FAV)-HOPE eye hospital. reproduced with permission.

3.1.3 Ocular motility alterations and vascular findings

Among infants with congenital Zika virus infection, the most commonly reported ocular motility disturbances include early-onset strabismus, nystagmus and ocular flutter [21, 25, 60]. The vascular findings are mainly subretinal hemorrhages and abnormalities in peripheral retinal vasculature, including abnormal termination of the retinal vessels, tortuosity and vascular attenuation [21].

3.1.4 Congenital glaucoma

This condition is rare (2.6%) but can occur in infants presenting with CZS and microcephaly. The related findings include and enlarged and cloudy cornea, buphthalmos, photophobia and excessive tearing [11, 57, 61].

The important increase in the prevalence of microcephaly in newborn infants in the Americas, in association with the previously described abnormal and vision-threatening ocular findings, should promptly lead to suspect the diagnosis of congenital infection due to Zika virus in these epidemic regions, which could be confirmed with real-time polymerase chain reaction in the first 5 days of acute phase of infection, after ruling out TORCH infections [62]. It is clear that infants with microcephaly should be screened for ocular lesions, but it is so important to consider that infants without microcephaly may have eye lesions. Then all children of the epidemic areas, such as South America, Central America and the Caribbean, with potential maternal Zika virus exposure at any time during pregnancy should be screened for ocular implication regardless of the presence of central nervous system alterations, because ocular findings could be underdiagnosed if microcephaly continues to be the main inclusion criterion in the screening of this group of children [16, 19, 63]. In addition, all newborns with mothers infected with Zika virus during pregnancy should have an early ophthalmological evaluation including the proper posterior pole examination through full dilation of the pupil [17, 64, 65].

3.2 Ocular findings in adults

The most important difference between infants and adults is that in adults there could be seen symptoms and signs of an active infectious process with the chance of detecting the Zika virus during a viremic period. In adults, only 20% of adults are symptomatic, and therefore the majority of adults with an acute Zika virus infection are asymptomatic [66]. Instead, in infants the related ocular findings are usually scars, as a manifestation of a post-infection process.

Symptomatic patients infected with Zika virus can exhibit a non-purulent conjunctivitis as a non-specific manifestation in the mild course of the disease [8, 67, 68]. Hypertensive iridocyclitis secondary to Zika virus infection has been reported during the acute phase of the disease, associated with ocular discomfort, redness and blurry vision, variable ciliary injection and anterior chamber reaction, miosis and elevation of the intraocular pressure. The findings usually ease after the viremia decreases and the use of topical treatment with steroids, cycloplegic and ocular hypotensive agents [69–71].

Other ocular findings in adults during acute infection include unilateral acute maculopathy, which exhibits a grayish annulus and pigment mottling as fundoscopic alterations, as well as disruption of the outer retinal and retinal pigment epithelium architecture in the central macula on optical coherence tomography and early hypofluorescence with irregular late central staining on angiogram, in addition to prompt resolution with visual function recovery [72, 73]. Neuroretinitis with a macular-star pattern has also been described in literature [74]. There could be found associated placoid or multifocal non-necrotizing chorioretinal lesions, especially in immunocompromised patients, that usually evolve with scaring and posterior improvement of visual acuity. Then, these chorioretinal lesions may be a manifestation of the active phase of infection in patients with viremia [24, 40, 75].

4. Systemic diagnosis

After clinical evaluation in individuals showing clinically compatible symptoms, the laboratory diagnosis of acute infection is based on the use of molecular tests for direct detection of viral nucleic acids (RNA) in blood and other biological samples and serological tests with tests of Enzymatic immunosorption (ELISA) or immunofluorescence assays (IFA) which allow the detection of IgM and IgG antibodies in serum. In a specialized manner, virus neutralization assays can also be performed to confirm the specificity of the ELISA or IFA tests, as well as cell cultures to isolate the virus [8, 76].

During the acute phase of the infection, the diagnosis is based on the detection of viral nucleic acid (RNA) by (RT-PCR) polymerase chain reaction of reverse transcription in blood, urine and saliva samples as well as in others biological samples such as CSF, amniotic fluid, semen [77], fetoplacental tissue and aqueous humor. Furtado et al. reported the case of a patient using aqueous humor to perform RT-PCR [70]. Two separate samples should be collected: the first during the acute phase and the second in the next 2–3 weeks [78]. If the result is negative, serological tests such as IGM should be supplemented, if they are positive, the plaque reduction neutralization test (PRNT) is performed as complement to determine whether or not there is a recent infection [76]. The conjunctival fluid contains virus for up to 7 days compared to urine and saliva samples of less than 20 days [79, 80].

4.1 Case confirmation

The Center for Disease Control recommends that an initial clinical evaluation should be performed in all infants with evidence of exposure to ZIKV or with suggestive laboratories, regardless of whether they have abnormalities consistent with ZIKV infection. There should be also evaluated those infants with abnormal clinical or neuroimaging findings, such as intracranial calcifications that were detected prenatally or during childbirth, and whose mothers were potentially infected with ZIKV during pregnancy [81].

According to the ECDC, a case is defined as confirmed when at least one of the following laboratory criteria is present: nucleic acid detection (RNA), antigens in a clinical sample; virus isolation in a clinical sample; detection of specific antibodies (IGM) in serum samples and confirmation by neutralization test; seroconversion or quadruple increase in the titer of specific antibodies against ZIKV in paired serum samples. A case is defined as probable if specific IgM antibodies are detected in serum. Epidemiological criteria must be taken into account [82]. It is recommended to perform funduscopy under pharmacological dilation in those patients with risk factors at least once within the first month and repeat at 3 months as a follow-up for those patients with confirmed diagnosis.

5. Ophthalmic diagnosis

ZIKV infection can occur with a wide spectrum of ocular findings, the most characteristic being the mottled pigment and chorioretinal atrophy that are commonly observed in the posterior pole especially in the macular area. There has been reported cases in the literature with manifestations that include conjunctivitis, uveitis [70], unilateral acute idiopathic maculopathy, chorioretinal lesions of acute onset, self-resolution, non-necrotizing multifocal placoids or manifestations such as manifestation of active chorioretinitis due to virus [75], optic neuropathy and congenital glaucoma [61], retinal vasculopathy [59], and hypertensive iridocyclitis [71].

The funduscopy is clinically important as a diagnostic tool and atrophic pigmented macular and peri-macular lesions, diffuse RPE damage and chorioretinal atrophy can be observed [14]. There are reports where funduscopy revealed pigmented external retinal lesions, retinal vascular abnormalities as tortuosity and dilation and atrophy of the optic nerve [11, 83]. In the peripheral retina a hypolucid spot can be observed as well as scattered subretinal hemorrhages external to the macula.

In fluorescein angiography early blockage and late staining in the retinal pigment epithelium is present. In autoflorescence, multimodal images showed a group of hyperautofluorescent lesions, it has also been described that there were focal areas of presumed choroiditis visualized as hypercynesic lesions in indocyanine green angiography [83].

Furtado et al. reported the case of a patient diagnosed with Zika by molecular and serological tests as well as positive ZIKV RNA in (RT-PCR) in aqueous humor obtained by anterior chamber paracentesis and described bilateral conjunctival hyperemia, bilateral non-granulomatous keratic precipitates and positive cellularity in the anterior chamber [70]. Parke et al. presented the case of a patient in whom alterations in the RPE with a gray ring around the fovea were observed and evidence by optical coherence tomography in the external retina and with macular area compromise. The above findings were in relation to a positive result for molecular testing with PRNT neutralization reduction technique of ZIKV [73].

5.1 Optical coherence tomography

For a better understanding of the ocular findings and as a follow-up to the characteristics probably related to ZIKV infection at the ocular level, some studies that analyzed the retinal tissue have been performed, Ventura et al. for example described the related findings by OCT in a series of consecutive cross-sectional cases that included 8 infants. The main OCT findings in the affected eyes included disruption of the ellipsoid zone and hyperreflectivity underlying the retinal pigment epithelium, thinning of the retina and choroid, and a colobomatous excavation [84].

Oliveira et al. described that the OCT results show a wide range of retinal damage caused by congenital ZIKV infection, and reinforced the findings compatible with chorioretinal atrophy [85]. Campos et al. described a case report with similar findings that correspond to retina thinning with atrophy of the external retina, including the outer nuclear layer and the ellipsoid zone, associated with hyperreflectivity of the RPE and increased OCT penetration into deeper layers of the choroid and sclera (**Figure 4**) [86].

Henry et al. used images of fluorescein-like fundus lesions and indocyanine green angiography, autofluorescence and optical coherence tomography associated with ZIKV and described acute and multifocal posterior non-necrotizing placoid epitheliopathy lesions that could be characteristic of active chorioretinitis due to ZIKV [75]. The findings described by OCT suggested that the neurotropism manifested by the ZIKV corresponds to significant necrosis areas of the retinal tissue.

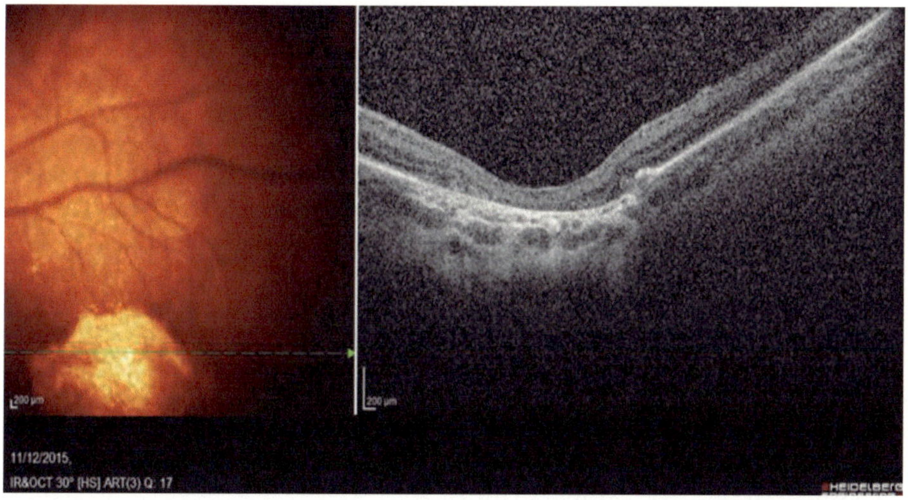

Figure 4.
Spectral domain OCT of a macular lesion in an infant with presumed Zika virus-associated microcephaly, demonstrating retinal thinning with atrophy of the outer retina, including the outer nuclear layer and ellipsoid zone, associated with retinal pigment epithelium hyper-reflectivity and increased penetration of OCT into deeper layers of the choroid and sclera. Taken from Campos AG, Lira RP, Arantes TE. Optical coherence tomography of macular atrophy associated with microcephaly and presumed intrauterine Zika virus infection. Arq bras Oftalmol. 2016;79(6):400–1. Reproduced with the permission from the author according to creative commons attribution license.

6. Systemic treatment

There is no specific approved antiviral treatment nor vaccines for the ZIKV infection to date. Actual treatment due to this virus is focused in control of symptoms (rest, fluid ingestion, antipyretics as paracetamol) [2, 53]. There are several compounds been tested in-vitro, each one with different action mechanism between each other's: Inhibition of the replication of the virus at early and late phases (For instance the Direct Acting Agents);inhibition of the molecular attachment, endocytosis and fusion mechanisms of the virus leading to block the viral entry, like duramycin, suramin and nanchangmycin [87, 88]. Some different molecules are being studied in animal models such as Z2 synthetic peptide inhibitor and the cholesterol-25-hydroxylase, which interfere vertical transmission in pregnant mice and cause cholesterol oxidation respectively [89, 90]. Novobioctin, lopinavir-ritonavir and bromocriptine cause an inhibition of the protease activity (NS2B-NS3 vial protease protein) [91, 92].

There is a growing interest in developing a vaccine against the ZIKV that could be used, especially in pregnant women. Animal models have been implemented, like knockout mice with shortcomings in IFN-I or IFN-II receptors, recreating many of the characteristics of the infection. The vaccine candidates that are been studied are in phase I or II, being the most promising a ZIKV-purified inactivate virus, or nucleic acid and adenovirus-based vaccines against the prM and E proteins providing long term protection in monkeys and mice [93–97].

7. Ocular treatment

There is no existence of guidelines or clinical trials about the treatment of ocular manifestation in ZIKV infection. The available data is extracted of case reports and case series. It is mandatory to focus the treatment according to the ophthalmic clinical context of each patient. In a patient with ophthalmologic manifestations that are presumed to be derived from ZIKV, it is necessary to exclude other causes before, then specific treatment is established.

In adults, ocular compromise in acute phases of the ZIKV infection could be treated with topical steroids, cycloplegic, and hypotensive topical medication according to ocular signs and symptoms present at that moment. Ocular compromise in children require a multidisciplinary approach and a focused treatment according to the present ocular conditions [53]. Cases with refractive errors, anisometropias, hypoaccomodation, amblyopia, and strabismus requires visual development therapies (eyeglasses, patching, ortoptics, and strabismus surgery) that are key in visual rehabilitation [12, 98].

Cases of anterior uveitis derived from ZIKV infection, usually are self-limiting course, which makes redundant the need of therapy [99]. However, there are cases of hypertensive acute anterior uveitis treated with β-Blockers and carbonic anhydrase inhibitor eyedrops accompanied or not with topical steroids and cycloplegics with normalization after treatment [70, 71, 100]. Kodati et al. reported an adult case of posterior uveitis and chorioretinal lesions in an inmunocompetent patient treated with loteprednol etabonate 0.5% three times daily, then reaching visual acuities of 20/20, with remaining photopsias [69].

Cases of bilateral optic neuritis in adults related to ZIKV were treated with intravenous methylprednisolone for 3 days followed by oral prednisolone for 11 additional days leading to a modest and partial recovery of visual acuity [61, 101]. Ocular flutter in a ZIKV post-infection state patient with neurological additional symptoms were described with improvement after intravenous immunoglobulin for 5 days [60].

Retinal disease associated to ZIKV, sometimes manifested as perifoveal microaneurysms with no involvement of visual function did not require any additional treatment beyond observation [59]. Acute maculopathy with bull's-eye shape were reported in an adult case, with total improvement of visual acuity after 6 weeks without any treatment [73]. There is a study were the pharmacological inhibition of ABCG1, a membrane transporter of cholesterol, resulted in reduced ZIKV infectivity of RPE [42].

Glaucoma in Congenital Zika syndrome is a visual-threatening condition that need special attention and early treatment, were the use of hypotensive topical medications and surgery like trabeculotomy, trabeculectomy, trabeculotomy plus trabeculectomy or goniotomy are the most used strategies [13, 21, 57, 61].

8. Visual prognosis in children with congenital ZIKV infection

The infants affected with congenital Zika virus syndrome may manifest many structural ocular findings in addition to the typical ones than involve the posterior pole, presenting low contrast sensitivity, visual field defects, hypoaccommodation, refractive errors and ocular motor disorders such as strabismus and nystagmus, commonly associated to neurological conditions, that finally interfere with the development of stereopsis and binocular vision. The sum of all of these findings results in severe visual impairment, regardless of the abnormalities of the retina and optic nerve [24].

There has been reported that even in the absence of apparent ocular abnormalities, there is a high prevalence of visual impairment between infants with microcephaly due to congenital Zika syndrome, suggesting that cerebral visual impairment, as a result of extensive damage to the central nervous system, could be the most frequent cause of blindness in affected infants [98, 102, 103]. This condition is known as cortical visual impairment, which is a reduction in visual response due to a neurologic issue. Then, the visual prognosis could be committed even in absence of ocular damage because of the severe cerebral malformation and abnormal brain development related to Zika infection. The affected infants usually have some vision and then they could exhibit improvement of their abilities over time. There could be seen the necessity of multidisciplinary teams for early cognitive and visual stimulation of newborns affected by congenital Zika virus syndrome, in order to decrease the impact of these infants and their families and achieve better quality of life. Further studies with long follow-up periods are needed to recognize the impact of the described ocular and neurological abnormalities, as well as for a better understanding and description of the natural history related to Zika infection and its ocular sequelae [13].

The early recognition, assessment and intervention of children with congenital Zika virus syndrome is crucial, especially in those ones that present hypoaccommodation and refractive errors, because they could show a significant improvement in visual acuity if they receive an early intervention with proper eyeglasses, as part of an integral visual stimulation therapy. For achieving significant changes in their refractive status it is necessary to guarantee periodical updates over time.

9. Visual prognosis in adults

In general terms, there is a benign visual evolution in adults, because the symptoms and signs are associated with a self-limited viral process related to the acute phase of Zika virus infection that usually resolves once the virus is cleared. Then, the vision returns to normal in the majority of the cases.

Non-purulent conjunctivitis is the most common non-congenital and self-limited ocular manifestation of Zika virus infection [101]. The adults that course with chorioretinal lesions, like immunocompromised patients that are in higher risk for presenting these fundus alterations, usually evolve as acute-onset and self-resolving lesions, with scaring and posterior improvement of visual acuity. Then this finding of Zika virus chorioretinitis may be a clear representation of the active phase of infection in a significant context of viremia. In the case of diagnosis of unilateral acute maculopathy related to Zika virus infection, the patient can be carefully monitored because there is usually visual function recovery, with improvement in the pigment epithelial and outer retinal architecture on optical coherence tomography after the acute illness [52].

There has been described many non-congenital ocular complications related to arboviral infection, including epiescleritis, keratitis, uveitis, vitritis, macular atrophy, retinal vascular occlusion, optic neuritis and macular edema, with no specific or pathognomonic ocular lesion for Zika virus infection. Most patients recover completely, but there is always a small percentage of patients that evolve with permanent damage and subsequently can lead to long-life visual impairment [65]. Uveitis can be identified in adults during active Zika virus infection and has a benign prognosis. It is considered the principal difference between the ocular manifestations seen in acquired Zika infection and those observed in congenital Zika virus syndrome, because uveitis has been only reported in the acquired cases during viremia. Most cases evolve to complete regression and recovery of visual acuity after the viremia decreases and the use of topical treatment with steroids, cycloplegic and ocular hypertension drops [12].

10. Conclusion

Ocular involvement by ZIKV is related to the ability to break the blood-retinal barrier and axonal transportation, leading to manifestations in children and adults.

Among the affected infants, the most common ophthalmologic manifestations include optic nerve hypoplasia, increased cup-to-disk ratio, macular scarring and focal pigmentary retinal mottling, as well as anterior ocular findings and ocular motility alterations. The most sever ophthalmic manifestations occur when the infection takes place in the first trimester of pregnancy, exposure to the virus during pregnancy can cause devastating effects on the developing fetus, specially affecting the central nervous system. The associated pattern of birth defects is known as congenital Zika virus syndrome among adults, the manifestations are usually self-limited and in some cases require some kind of treatment. It is needed to focus the treatment according to the ophthalmic clinical context of each patient. Cases with CZS should be enrolled in an integral and multidisciplinary team for providing early-intervention services including cognitive and visual rehabilitation. Further studies are necessary to recognize the impact of ocular damage and neurological abnormalities and its long-term consequences in the affected children.

Acknowledgements

The authors thank Camila Ventura, MD, PhD from Altino Ventura Foundation (FAV) and HOPE Eye Hospital, and Adriana Gondim de Moura Campos from Universida de Federal de Pernambuco for having provided images from their daily clinical practice and previous works, being a great complement to this chapter.

Author details

Dayron Fernando Martínez-Pulgarín[1,2,3*], Carlos Miguel Córdoba-Ortega[1,2] and Fabio Daniel Padilla-Pantoja[1,2]

1 Department of Ophthalmology, School of Medicine, Universidad Nacional de Colombia, Bogota, Colombia

2 Basic and Clinic Ophthalmology Research Group, School of Medicine, Universidad Nacional de Colombia, Bogota, Colombia

3 Research Group and Incubator Public Health and Infection, Faculty of Health Sciences, Universidad Tecnológica de Pereira, Pereira, Colombia

*Address all correspondence to: dayronfernando@hotmail.com

References

[1] Dick G, Kitchen SF, Haddow A. Zika virus (I). Isolations and serological specificity. Transactions of the Royal Society of Tropical Medicina and Hygiene. 1952;**45**(5):509-520

[2] Ferraris P, Yssel H, Misse D. Zika virus infection: An update. Microbes and Infection. 2019

[3] Martinez-Pulgarin DF, Acevedo-Mendoza WF, Cardona-Ospina JA, Rodriguez-Morales AJ, Paniz-Mondolfi AE. A bibliometric analysis of global Zika research. Travel Medicine and Infectious Disease. 2016;**14**(1):55-57

[4] Rodríguez-Morales AJ, Trujillo AM, Sánchez-Duque JA, Cardona-OspinaJA, Villamil-GómezWE, Jimenez-Canizalez CE, et al. Introductory Chapter: Clinical and Epidemiological Implications of Zika Virus Infection - The Experience of RECOLZIKA in Colombia; 2018

[5] Pinazo-Duran MD, Silva ED. Zika virus. A teratogenic agent for the eyes. Archivos de la Sociedad Española de Oftalmología. 2017;**92**(2):51-53

[6] Benzekri R, Belfort R Jr, Ventura CV, de Paula FB, Maia M, Leite M, et al. Ocular manifestations of Zika virus: What we do and do not know. Journal Français d'Ophtalmologie. 2017;**40**(2):138-145

[7] de Andrade GC, Ventura CV, Mello Filho PA, Maia M, Vianello S, Rodrigues EB. Arboviruses and the eye. International Journal of Retina and Vitreous. 2017;**3**:4

[8] Sahiner F, Sig AK, Savasci U, Tekin K, Akay F. Zika virus-associated ocular and neurologic disorders: The emergence of new evidence. The Pediatric Infectious Disease Journal. 2017;**36**(12):e341-e3e6

[9] Buathong R, Hermann L, Thaisomboonsuk B, Rutvisuttinunt W, Klungthong C, Chinnawirotpisan P, et al. Detection of Zika virus infection in Thailand, 2012-2014. The American Journal of Tropical Medicine and Hygiene. 2015;**93**(2):380-383

[10] Nithiyanantham SF, Badawi A. Maternal infection with Zika virus and prevalence of congenital disorders in infants: Systematic review and meta-analysis. Canadian Journal of Public Health. 2019

[11] de Paula FB, Ventura CV, Maia M, Belfort R Jr. Zika virus and the eye. Current Opinion in Ophthalmology. 2017;**28**(6):595-599

[12] Ventura C, Ventura LO. Ophthalmologic manifestations associated with Zika virus infection. Pediatrics. 2018;**141**(s2):S161-S166

[13] de Oliveira Dias JR, Ventura CV, de Paula FB, Prazeres J, Ventura LO, Bravo-Filho V, et al. Ocular abnormalities in congenital Zika syndrome: Are the ophthalmoscopic findings "the top of the iceberg"? Progress in Retinal and Eye Research. 2018;**66**:85-106

[14] Ventura CV, Maia M, Bravo-Filho V, Góis AL, Belfort R. Zika virus in Brazil and macular atrophy in a child with microcephaly. The Lancet. 2016;**387**(10015):228

[15] Ventura CV, Maia M, Ventura BV, Linden VV, Araujo EB, Ramos RC, et al. Ophthalmological findings in infants with microcephaly and presumable intra-uterus Zika virus infection. Arquivos Brasileiros de Oftalmologia. 2016;**79**(1):1-3

[16] Ventura CV, Maia M, Dias N, Ventura LO, Belfort R. Zika: Neurological and ocular findings in

infant without microcephaly. The Lancet. 2016;**387**(10037):2502

[17] de Paula FB, de Oliveira Dias JR, Prazeres J, Sacramento GA, Ko AI, Maia M, et al. Ocular findings in infants with microcephaly associated with presumed Zika virus congenital infection in Salvador, Brazil. JAMA Ophthalmology. 2016;**134**(5):529-535

[18] Vercosa I, Carneiro P, Vercosa R, Girao R, Ribeiro EM, Pessoa A, et al. The visual system in infants with microcephaly related to presumed congenital Zika syndrome. Journal of AAPOS. 2017;**21**(4):300-304.e1

[19] Zin AA, Tsui I, Rossetto J, Vasconcelos Z, Adachi K, Valderramos S, et al. Screening criteria for ophthalmic manifestations of congenital Zika virus infection. JAMA Pediatrics. 2017;**171**(9):847-854

[20] Acosta-Reyes J, Navarro E, Herrera MJ, Goenaga E, Ospina ML, Parra E, et al. Severe neurologic disorders in 2 fetuses with Zika virus infection, Colombia. Emerging Infectious Diseases. 2017;**23**(6):982-984

[21] Yepez JB, Murati FA, Pettito M, Penaranda CF, de Yepez J, Maestre G, et al. Ophthalmic manifestations of congenital Zika syndrome in Colombia and Venezuela. JAMA Ophthalmology. 2017;**135**(5):440-445

[22] Alvarado-Socarras JL, Aux-Cadena CP, Murillo-Garcia DR, Rodriguez-Morales AJ. Ophthalmologic evaluation in infants of mothers with Zika: A report from Colombia. Travel Medicine and Infectious Disease. 2019

[23] Ventura CV, Maia M, Travassos SB, Martins TT, Patriota F, Nunes ME, et al. Risk factors associated with the Ophthalmoscopic findings identified in infants with presumed Zika virus congenital infection. JAMA Ophthalmology. 2016;**134**(8):912-918

[24] Ventura CV, Ventura Filho MC, Ventura LO. Ocular manifestations and visual outcome in children with congenital Zika syndrome. Topics in Magnetic Resonance Imaging. 2019;**28**(1):23-27

[25] Baran LCP, da Costa MF, Vidal KS, Damico FM, Barboni MTS, da SLD, et al. Alterations in visual acuity and visual development in infants 1-24 months old either exposed to or infected by Zika virus during gestation, with and without microcephaly. Journal of AAPOS. 2019;**23**:215.e1-215.e7

[26] Chan JF, Choi GK, Yip CC, Cheng VC, Yuen KY. Zika fever and congenital Zika syndrome: An unexpected emerging arboviral disease. The Journal of Infection. 2016;**72**(5):507-524

[27] Smith DR, Sprague TR, Hollidge BS, Valdez SM, Padilla SL, Bellanca SA, et al. African and Asian Zika virus isolates display phenotypic differences both In vitro and In vivo. The American Journal of Tropical Medicine and Hygiene. 2018;**98**(2):432-444

[28] Hajra A, Bandyopadhyay D, Hajra SK. Zika virus: A global threat to humanity: A comprehensive review and current developments. North American Journal of Medical Sciences. 2016;**8**(3):123-128

[29] Salinas S, Foulongne V, Loustalot F, Fournier-Wirth C, Moles JP, Briant L, et al. [Zika virus, an emerging threat]. Medical Science (Paris). 2016;32(4):378-386

[30] Calvet G, Aguiar RS, Melo ASO, Sampaio SA, de Filippis I, Fabri A, et al. Detection and sequencing of Zika virus from amniotic fluid of fetuses with microcephaly in Brazil: A case study. The Lancet Infectious Diseases. 2016;**16**(6):653-660

[31] Martines RB, Bhatnagar J, Keating MK, Silva-Flannery L, Muehlenbachs A, Gary J, et al. Evidence of Zika virus infection in brain and placental tissues from two congenitally infected newborns and two fetal losses — Brazil, 2015. Morbidity and Mortality Weekly Report. 2015;**65**:159-160

[32] Motta IJ, Spencer BR, Cordeiro da Silva SG, Arruda MB, Dobbin JA, Gonzaga YB, et al. Evidence for transmission of Zika virus by platelet transfusion. Obstetric Anesthesia Digest. 2017;**37**(1):53

[33] Slenczka W. Zika virus disease. Microbiology Spectrum. 2016;**4**:163-173

[34] de Paula FB, Zin A, Ko A, Maia M, Ventura CV, Belfort R Jr. Anterior-segment ocular findings and microphthalmia in congenital Zika syndrome. Ophthalmology. 2017;**124**(12):1876-1878

[35] Fernandez MP, Parra Saad E, Ospina Martinez M, Corchuelo S, Mercado Reyes M, Herrera MJ, et al. Ocular histopathologic features of congenital Zika syndrome. JAMA Ophthalmology. 2017;**135**(11): 1163-1169

[36] Pandey RK, Yu F-S, Kumar A. Targeting toll-like receptor signaling as a novel approach to prevent ocular infectious diseases. The Indian Journal of Medical Research. 2013;**138**(5):609-619

[37] Constable PA, Lawrenson JG. Glial cell factors and the outer blood retinal barrier. Ophthalmic & Physiological Optics. 2009;**29**(5):557-564

[38] Rossi SL, Tesh RB, Azar SR, Muruato AE, Hanley KA, Auguste AJ, et al. Characterization of a novel murine model to study Zika virus. The American Journal of Tropical Medicine and Hygiene. 2016;**94**(6):1362-1369

[39] Dowall SD, Graham VA, Rayner E, Atkinson B, Hall G, Watson RJ, et al. A susceptible mouse model for Zika virus infection. PLoS Neglected Tropical Diseases. 2016;**10**(5):e0004658

[40] Manangeeswaran M, Kielczewski JL, Sen HN, Xu BC, Ireland DDC, McWilliams IL, et al. ZIKA virus infection causes persistent chorioretinal lesions. Emerging Microbes & Infections. 2018;**7**(1):96

[41] Roach T, Alcendor DJ. Zika virus infection of cellular components of the blood-retinal barriers: Implications for viral associated congenital ocular disease. Journal of Neuroinflammation. 2017;**14**(1):43

[42] Singh PK, Khatri I, Jha A, Pretto CD, Spindler KR, Arumugaswami V, et al. Determination of system level alterations in host transcriptome due to Zika virus (ZIKV) infection in retinal pigment epithelium. Scientific Reports. 2018;**8**(1):11209

[43] Singh PK, Kasetti RB, Zode GS, Goyal A, Juzych MS, Kumar A. Zika virus infects trabecular meshwork and causes trabeculitis and glaucomatous pathology in mouse eyes. mSphere. 2019;**4**(3):1-14

[44] Miner JJ, Sene A, Richner JM, Smith AM, Santeford A, Ban N, et al. Zika virus infection in mice causes panuveitis with shedding of virus in tears. Cell Reports. 2016;**16**(12):3208-3218

[45] van den Pol AN, Mao G, Yang Y, Ornaghi S, Davis JN. Zika virus targeting in the developing brain. The Journal of Neuroscience. 2017;**37**(8): 2161-2175

[46] Singh PK, Guest JM, Kanwar M, Boss J, Gao N, Juzych MS, et al. Zika virus infects cells lining the blood-retinal barrier and causes chorioretinal atrophy in mouse eyes. JCI Insight. 2017;**2**(4):e92340

[47] Zhao Z, Yang M, Azar SR, Soong L, Weaver SC, Sun J, et al. Viral retinopathy in experimental models of Zika infection. Investigative Ophthalmology & Visual Science. 2017;**58**(10):4355-4365

[48] Aleman TS, Ventura CV, Cavalcanti MM, Serrano LW, Traband A, Nti AA, et al. Quantitative assessment of microstructural changes of the retina in infants with congenital Zika syndrome. JAMA Ophthalmology. 2017;**135**(10):1069-1076

[49] Miranda HA 2nd, Costa MC, Frazao MAM, Simao N, Franchischini S, Moshfeghi DM. Expanded spectrum of congenital ocular findings in microcephaly with presumed Zika infection. Ophthalmology. 2016;**123**(8):1788-1794

[50] Prakalapakorn SG, Meaney-Delman D, Honein MA, Rasmussen SA. The eyes as a window to improved understanding of the prenatal effects of Zika virus infection. Journal of AAPOS. 2017;**21**(4):259-261

[51] Valentine G, Marquez L, Pammi M. Zika virus-associated microcephaly and eye lesions in the newborn. Journal of the Pediatric Infectious Diseases Society. 2016;**5**(3):323-328

[52] Guevara JG, Agarwal-Sinha S. Ocular abnormalities in congenital Zika syndrome: A case report, and review of the literature. Journal of Medical Case Reports. 2018;**12**(1):161

[53] Marquezan MC, Ventura CV, Sheffield JS, Golden WC, Omiadze R, Belfort R Jr, et al. Ocular effects of Zika virus-a review. Survey of Ophthalmology. 2018;**63**(2):166-173

[54] Tang H, Hammack C, Ogden SC, Wen Z, Qian X, Li Y, et al. Zika virus infects human cortical neural progenitors and attenuates their growth. Cell Stem Cell. 2016;**18**(5):587-590

[55] Faizan MI, Abdullah M, Ali S, Naqvi IH, Ahmed A, Parveen S. Zika virus-induced microcephaly and its possible molecular mechanism. Intervirology. 2016;**59**(3):152-158

[56] Calle-Giraldo JP, Rojas CA, Hurtado IC, Barco C, Libreros D, Sanchez PJ, et al. Outcomes of congenital Zika virus infection during an outbreak in Valle Del Cauca, Colombia. The Pediatric Infectious Disease Journal. 2019;**38**(7):735-740

[57] de Oliveira DR, Ventura CV, Esporcatte BLB, Gracitelli CPB, Dias NC, Ventura LO, et al. Glaucoma workup in congenital Zika syndrome. Journal of Glaucoma. 2019;**28**(4):313-317

[58] Gely-RojasL, PérezR, García-FragosoL, García-García I. Association of Zika virus exposure in utero with ocular phenotypes in a group of newborns in Puerto Rico. Puerto Rico Health Sciences Journal. 2018;**37**:s77-s80

[59] Singh MS, Marquezan MC, Omiadze R, Reddy AK, Belfort R Jr, May WN. Inner retinal vasculopathy in Zika virus disease. American Journal of Ophthalmology Case Reports. 2018;**10**:6-7

[60] Karam E, Giraldo J, Rodriguez F, Hernandez-Pereira CE, Rodriguez-Morales AJ, Blohm GM, et al. Ocular flutter following Zika virus infection. Journal of Neurovirology. 2017;**23**(6):932-934

[61] De Moraes CG, Pettito M, Yepez JB, Sakuntabhai A, Simon-Loriere E, Zaidi MB, et al. Optic neuropathy and congenital glaucoma associated with probable Zika virus infection in Venezuelan patients. JMM Case Report. 2018;**5**(5):e005145

[62] Jurgens I, Rey A. Ocular findings in patients with microcephaly can suggest presumed congenital zika virus infection. Acta Ophthalmologica. 2018;**96**(4):423-424

[63] Ventura CV, Fernandez MP, Gonzalez IA, Rivera-Hernandez DM, Lopez-Alberola R, Peinado M, et al. First travel-associated congenital zika syndrome in the US: Ocular and neurological findings in the absence of microcephaly. Ophthalmic Surgery, Lasers & Imaging Retina. 2016;**47**(10):952-955

[64] Bandyopadhyay D, Hajra A. ZIKA virus: A new threat to the eyes. European Journal of Internal Medicine. 2017;**44**:e9-e10

[65] McCarthy M. Severe eye damage in infants with microcephaly is presumed to be due to Zika virus. BMJ. 2016;**352**:i855

[66] Centers for Disease Control and Prevention NCfEaZIDN, Division of Vector-Borne Diseases (DVBD). About Zika. 2019. Available from: https://www.cdc.gov/zika/about/index.html

[67] Agrawal R, Oo HH, Balne PK, Ng L, Tong L, Leo YS. Zika virus and the eye. Ocular Immunology and Inflammation. 2018;**26**(5):654-659

[68] Platt DJ, Miner JJ. Consequences of congenital Zika virus infection. Current Opinion in Virology. 2017;**27**:1-7

[69] Kodati S, Palmore TN, Spellman FA, Cunningham D, Weistrop B, Sen HN. Bilateral posterior uveitis associated with Zika virus infection. The Lancet. 2017;**389**(10064):125-126

[70] Furtado JM, Esposito DL, Klein TM, Teixeira-Pinto T, da Fonseca BA. Uveitis associated with Zika virus infection. The New England Journal of Medicine. 2016;**375**(4):394-396

[71] Fontes BM. Zika virus-related hypertensive iridocyclitis. Arquivos Brasileiros de Oftalmologia. 2016;**79**(1):63

[72] Wong C, Ng S, Cheung C, Wong T, Mathur R. Zika-related maculopathy. Retinal Cases & Brief Reports. 2017:1-3

[73] Parke DW 3rd, Almeida DR, Albini TA, Ventura CV, Berrocal AM, Mittra RA. Serologically confirmed Zika-related unilateral acute maculopathy in an adult. Ophthalmology. 2016;**123**(11):2432-2433

[74] Panday A, Sandy S, King D, Ramdeen S. A case of suspected symptomatic Zika neuroretinitis. IDCases. 2017;**9**:104-105

[75] Henry CR, Al-Attar L, Cruz-Chacon AM, Davis JL. Chorioretinal lesions presumed secondary to Zika virus infection in an immunocompromised adult. JAMA Ophthalmology. 2017;**135**(4):386-389

[76] Barzon L, Trevisan M, Sinigaglia A, Lavezzo E, Palù G. Zika virus: From pathogenesis to disease control. FEMS Microbiology Letters. 2016;**363**(18):1-17

[77] Sikka V, Chattu V, Popli R, Galwankar S, Kelkar D, Sawicki S, et al. The emergence of zika virus as a global health security threat: A review and a consensus statement of the INDUSEM joint working group (JWG). Journal of Global Infectious Diseases. 2016;**8**(1):3-15

[78] Hayes EB. Zika virus outside Africa. Emerging Infectious Diseases. 2009;**15**(9):1347-1350

[79] Adebanjo T, Godfred-Cato S, Viens L, Fischer M, Staples E, Kuhnert-Tallman W. Update: Interim guidance for the diagnosis, evaluation, and Management of Infants with possible congenital Zika virus infection — United States, October

2017. MMWR. Morbidity and Mortality Weekly Report. 2017;**66**(41):1089-1099

[80] Sun J, Wu D, Zhong H, Guan D, Zhang H, Tan Q, et al. Presence of Zika virus in Conjunctival fluid. JAMA Ophthalmology. 2016;**134**(11):1330-1332

[81] Hazin AN, Poretti A, Turchi CM, Huisman TA. Computed tomographic findings in microcephaly associated with Zika virus. The New England Journal of Medicine. 2016;**374**(22):2192-2193

[82] Control. ECfDPa. Interim guidance for healthcare providers and Zika virus laboratory diagnosis. Stockholm; 2016

[83] Ahmad SS, Amin TN, Ustianowski A. Zika virus: Management of infection and risk. BMJ. 2016;**352**:i1062

[84] Ventura CV, Ventura LO, Bravo-Filho V, Martins TT, Berrocal AM, Gois AL, et al. Optical coherence tomography of retinal lesions in infants with congenital Zika syndrome. JAMA Ophthalmology. 2016;**134**(12):1420-1427

[85] de Oliveira Dias JR, Ventura CV, Borba PD, de Paula FB, Pierroti LC, do Nascimento AP, et al. Infants with congenital zika syndrome and ocular findings from São Paulo, Brazil: Spread of infection. Retinal Cases and Brief Reports. 2018;**12**(4):382-386

[86] Campos AG, Lira RP, Arantes TE. Optical coherence tomography of macular atrophy associated with microcephaly and presumed intrauterine Zika virus infection. Arquivos Brasileiros de Oftalmologia. 2016;**79**(6):400-401

[87] Rausch K, Hackett BA, Weinbren NL, Reeder SM, Sadovsky Y, Hunter CA, et al. Screening bioactives reveals Nanchangmycin as a broad Spectrum antiviral active against Zika virus. Cell Reports. 2017;**18**(3):804-815

[88] Albulescu IC, Kovacikova K, Tas A, Snijder EJ, van Hemert MJ. Suramin inhibits Zika virus replication by interfering with virus attachment and release of infectious particles. Antiviral Research. 2017;**143**:230-236

[89] Yu Y, Deng YQ, Zou P, Wang Q, Dai Y, Yu F, et al. A peptide-based viral inactivator inhibits Zika virus infection in pregnant mice and fetuses. Nature Communications. 2017;**8**:15672

[90] Li C, Deng YQ, Wang S, Ma F, Aliyari R, Huang XY, et al. 25-Hydroxycholesterol protects host against Zika virus infection and its associated microcephaly in a mouse model. Immunity. 2017;**46**(3):446-456

[91] Yuan S, Chan JF, den-Haan H, Chik KK, Zhang AJ, Chan CC, et al. Structure-based discovery of clinically approved drugs as Zika virus NS2B-NS3 protease inhibitors that potently inhibit Zika virus infection in vitro and in vivo. Antiviral Research. 2017;**145**:33-43

[92] Chan JF, Chik KK, Yuan S, Yip CC, Zhu Z, Tee KM, et al. Novel antiviral activity and mechanism of bromocriptine as a Zika virus NS2B-NS3 protease inhibitor. Antiviral Research. 2017;**141**:29-37

[93] Poland GA, Kennedy RB, Ovsyannikova IG, Palacios R, Ho PL, Kalil J. Development of vaccines against Zika virus. The Lancet Infectious Diseases. 2018;**18**(7):e211-e219

[94] Abbink P, Stephenson KE, Barouch DH. Zika virus vaccines. Nature Reviews. Microbiology. 2018;**16**(10):594-600

[95] Masmejan S, Baud D, Musso D, Panchaud A. Zika virus, vaccines, and antiviral strategies. Expert

Review of Anti-Infective Therapy. 2018;**16**(6):471-483

[96] Larocca RA, Abbink P, Peron JP, Zanotto PM, Iampietro MJ, Badamchi-Zadeh A, et al. Vaccine protection against Zika virus from Brazil. Nature. 2016;**536**(7617):474-478

[97] Xu K, Song Y, Dai L, Zhang Y, Lu X, Xie Y, et al. Recombinant chimpanzee adenovirus vaccine AdC7-M/E protects against Zika virus infection and testis damage. Journal of Virology. 2018;**92**(6):1-16

[98] Ventura LO, Lawrence L, Ventura CV, Dutton GN, Marinho P, Ferro PF, et al. Response to correction of refractive errors and hypoaccommodation in children with congenital Zika syndrome. Journal of AAPOS. 2017;**21**(6):480-484.e1

[99] Zandi S, Bodaghi B, Garweg JG. Review for disease of the year: Treatment of viral anterior uveitis: A perspective. Ocular Immunology and Inflammation. 2018;**26**(7):1135-1142

[100] Merle H, Najioullah F, Chassery M, Césaire R, Hage R. Zika-related bilateral hypertensive anterior acute uveitis. JAMA Ophthalmology. 2017;**135**(3):283-284

[101] Zaidi MB, De Moraes CG, Petitto M, Yepez JB, Sakuntabhai A, Simon-Loriere E, et al. Non-congenital severe ocular complications of Zika virus infection. JMM Case Report. 2018;**5**(6):e005152

[102] Ventura LO, Ventura CV, Dias NC, Vilar IG, Gois AL, Arantes TE, et al. Visual impairment evaluation in 119 children with congenital Zika syndrome. Journal of AAPOS. 2018;**22**(3):218-222 e1

[103] Ventura LO, Ventura CV, Lawrence L, van der Linden V, van der Linden A, Gois AL, et al. Visual impairment in children with congenital Zika syndrome. Journal of AAPOS. 2017;**21**(4):295-299.e2

Section 3

Zika and Guillain-Barré Syndrome

Chapter 6

Guillain-Barre Syndrome and Miller Fisher Variant in Zika Virus Disease

Raafat Hammad Seroor Jadah

Abstract

Guillain-Barre syndrome (GBS) is a serious neurological disorder associated with a rapid progressive ascending muscle paralysis, and it is the most common neurological autoimmune disorder that affects the peripheral nervous system, which is usually triggered by viral or bacterial infection. GBS is rare in children and characterized by rapid progressive onset ascending muscle weakness associated with pain and sensory dysfunction. Miller Fisher syndrome (MFS), a variant of GBS, is rare in pediatric population which is typically manifested by ataxic gait, ophthalmoplegia, and areflexia since it is rare in children. It is vitally important to early diagnose this condition and to initiate early treatment to prevent further complications and long-term morbidity. Since the outbreak of Zika virus, the incidence of GBS has been increased. Zika virus associated with autoimmune anti-ganglioside antibodies trigger which lead to GBS development. Zika virus infection should be strongly considered in patients who present with classical signs of Miller Fisher syndrome, especially travelers and residents from endemic areas.

Keywords: Guillain-Barre, Miller Fisher, autoimmune, Zika, outbreak, ataxia

1. Introduction

1.1 History

In 1916, two French Neurologists Georges Charles Guillain and Jean Alexandre Barre and French Physiologist Andre Strohl reported an original paper encountered new syndrome in two soldiers with muscle weakness, absence of deep tendon reflexes and sensory impairment and described the key diagnosis of albumin-cytologic disassociation in the cerebrospinal fluid along with changes in electromyography and nerve conduction studies. Both patients were managed with massage therapy and Strychnine injection and showed clinical recovery after few months [1].

GBS is rare but the commonest cause for acute ascending paralytic polynephropathy. GBS is considered to be an acute immune-mediated disorder that causes peripheral polyneuropathy. Most cases of GBS are preceded by either viral or bacterial infection, which triggers the immune system affecting the peripheral nervous system causing a rapid progressive demyelinating polyneuropathy [2, 3].

The incidence of GBS has been increased since the outbreak of certain infections such as Zika virus epidemic in Latin America in 2015. GBS is the most leading cause of acute ascending muscle paralysis with an annual incidence of 1–2 per 100,000 persons per year worldwide. GBS is more common in males than females [2, 3].

GBS is a rapid demyelinating peripheral neuropathy that typically manifest as ascending muscle weakness that is symmetric in nature associated with reduced or absent deep tendon reflexes. GBS has been also associated with pain along with sensory impairment [4].

GBS is an acute immune-mediated demyelinating polyneuropathy and it is the commonest cause of acute muscle paralysis in pediatric age group patients [5, 6].

MFS is a rare neurological disorder which was initially recognized in 1932 by James Collier as a classical triad of ophthalmoplegia, ataxia and absent deep tendon reflexes. Later in 1956 Charles Miller Fisher a Canadian Neurologist described and reported details isolated clinical entity of three patients who presented with ophthalmoplegia, ataxia and areflexia [7].

MFS has an annual incidence of 0.9 per 1000,000 populations and affect males more than females at ratio of 2:1 and commonly affect Asian population especially at their fourth decade of life [7].

MFS most commonly preceded by *Campylobacter jejuni* infection and has strong association with positive anti-GQ1b antibodies [7].

Zika virus infection has been associated with different neurological disorders such as microcephaly and since the initial outbreak of Zika virus infection the number of GBS cases has been increased in endemic countries [8].

2. Pathophysiology and immunopathology

The neurological symptoms and signs of GBS usually take place 4 weeks after the initial respiratory or gastrointestinal infection which account for about

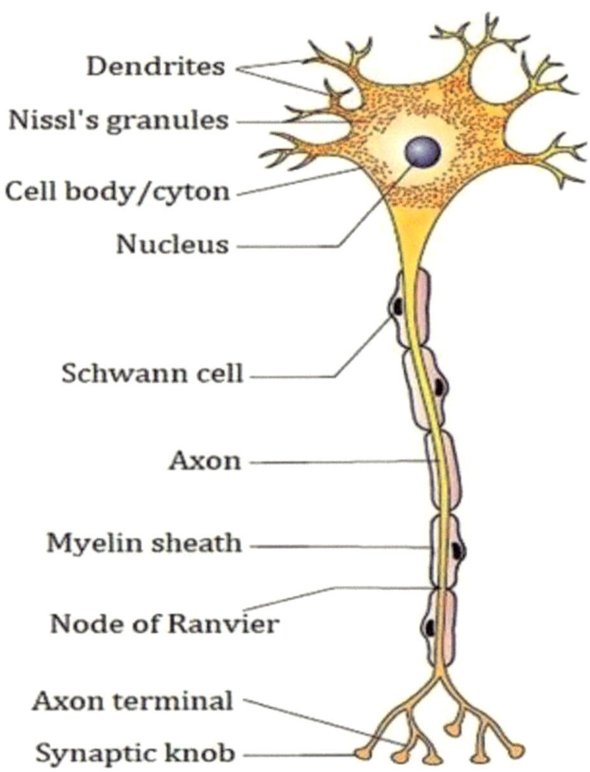

Figure 1.
Basic structure of motor neuron [10].

two-third of GBS cases in adult population. The immune system will be stimulated secondary to infectious antigen with *Campylobacter jejuni* (*C. jejuni*) being the most common infectious pathogenic agent which account for 25–50% of adult GBS cases [9]. These infectious antigens cause stimulation of both cellular and hormonal systems leading to axonal damage and demyelination of the peripheral nerve and nerve roots (**Figure 1**) [11].

Monocytes, T-cells, especially CD4+ T-helper cells and B-cells in order of frequency, have been commonly implicated in the immunopathology of GBS cases especially in the acute inflammatory demyelinating polyradiculoneuropathy (AIDP) [11].

More than 80% of the patients with Miller Fisher syndrome have anti-GQ1b IgG antibodies which mainly activate the compliment system especially at the presynaptic nerve ending and perisynaptic Schwann cells which has been implicated in the pathogenesis of MFS [11, 12].

3. Clinical features

GBS is a rapid inflammatory ascending symmetric muscle weakness associated with reduced or complete absent of deep tendon reflexes. The most common symptom is inability to walk. The frequent findings on the clinical examination include hyperesthesia, autonomic dysfunction, sensory loss, ataxia, bilateral facial nerve palsy and third cranial nerve palsy [4, 13].

3.1 Clinical subtypes of Guillain-Barre syndrome (GBS)

A number of clinical subtypes of Guillain-Barre Syndrome (GBS) are identified.

Acute inflammatory demyelinating polyradiculoneuropathy (AIDP) is considered to be the most common subtype and account for approximately of 90 percent of GBS patients in the Unites States. Patients with this subtype typically present with progressive ascending symmetric muscle weakness and areflexia associated with severe pain and autonomic dysfunction such as fluctuation in blood pressure, urinary incontinence or syncope. This clinical subtype typically shows a slow nerve conduction velocity with no clear anti-ganglioside antibodies association [14].

Other subtype of GBS is the acute motor axonal neuropathy (AMAN) that accounts for 5% of Guillain-Barre syndrome (GBS) patients in United States. This subtype purely presents with motor weakness without sensory symptoms. Nerve conduction study shows axonal polyneuropathy with normal sensory nerve action potential. Patients with acute motor axonal motor neuropathy have strong association with *Campylobacter jejuni* (*C. jejuni*) infection with positive antibodies against gangliosides GM1, GD1a, GalNac-GD1a and GD1b [14].

The acute motor-sensory axonal neuropathy (AMSAN) is a rare and severe variant of GBS [15], which has similar clinical features to acute motor axonal neuropathy but with predominantly sensory loss and positive antibodies against GM1 and GD1a. Nerve conduction study showed axonal polyneuropathy with reduced or absent sensory nerve action potential [14].

The pharyngeal-cervical brachial syndrome (PCB) is another rare subtype of GBS [16]. Patient with PCB syndrome typically present with rapid and progressive oropharyngeal and shoulder muscle weakness associated with absent deep tendon reflexes in the upper limbs. The nerve conduction study in patients with PCB syndrome is generally normal but sometimes showed axonal neuropathy in the arms. PCB syndrome associated with positive IgG anti-GT1a antibodies [17].

Miller Fisher syndrome is one of the GBS variant. It is an uncommon neurological disorder which account of about 5% of GBS cases. Patients with Miller Fisher syndrome typically present with clinical trial of ophthalmoplegia which is bilateral symmetric in most patients, ataxia and absent deep tendon reflexes. The commonest initial presenting symptoms in patients with Miller Fisher syndrome is diplopia (double vision) which is due to acute onset-ophthalmoplegia. Other less frequent signs and symptoms of MFS include headache, difficulty swallowing and photophobia (**Table 1**). MFS is an immune-mediated neurological disorder and more than 80% of patients with MFS showed positive IgG anti-GQ1b antibodies. Electrophysiological findings in patients with MFS commonly showed reduced sensory nerve action potentials and absent H reflexes (**Figure 2** and **Table 2**) [7, 12, 18].

Bickerstaff brainstem encephalitis currently considered to be another variant of Fisher syndrome associated with central nervous system involvement. Patients with Bickerstaff brainstem encephalitis typically present with ophthalmoplegia, ataxia, hyperreflexia and altered sensorium [19].

Bickerstaff brainstem encephalitis is an immune-mediated neurological disorder usually preceded by infection and associated with positive anti-GQ1b antibodies [19].

• Double vision (diplopia): most common
• Abnormal gait (ataxia)
• **Less frequent symptoms**
• Headache
• Difficulty swallowing (dysphagia)
• Light intolerance (photophobia)

Table 1.
Clinical symptoms associated with MFS.

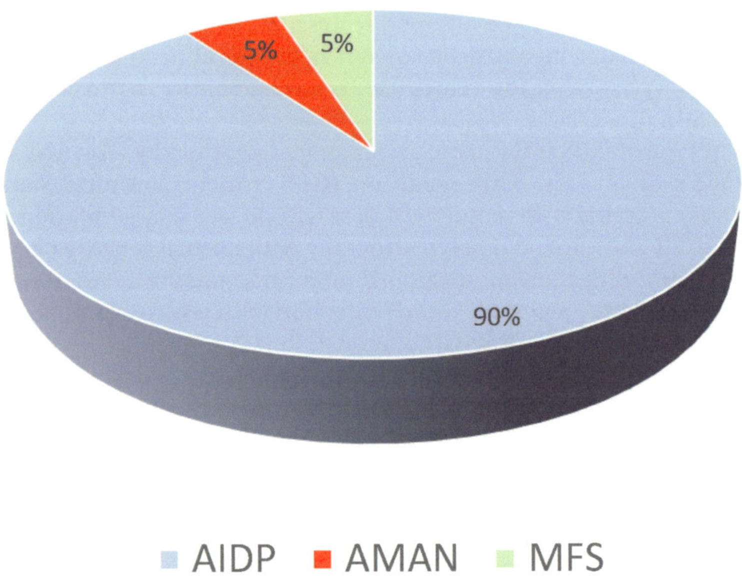

Figure 2.
Percentage of different subtypes of GBS [14, 18].

Type	Clinical symptoms	Electrophysiological findings	Serological tests
Acute inflammatory demyelinating polyradiculoneuropathy	Muscle weakness with sensory and autonomic dysfunction	Slow nerve conduction velocity	No clear anti-ganglioside antibodies association
Acute motor axonal neuropathy	Muscle weakness with no sensory impairment	Axonal polyneuropathy with normal sensory nerve action potential	Positive anti-ganglioside antibodies GM1, GD1a, GalNac-GD1a, and GD1b
Acute motor-sensory axonal neuropathy	Muscle weakness with sensory involvement	Axonal polyneuropathy with absent or reduced sensory nerve action potential	Positive antibodies against GM1 and GD1a
Pharyngeal-cervical brachial variant	Oropharyngeal and shoulder muscle weakness	Generally normal, occasional axonal neuropathy in the arms	Positive IgG anti-GT1a antibodies
Miller Fisher syndrome	Ophthalmoplegia, ataxia and areflexia	Reduced sensory nerve action potential and absent H-reflexes	Positive IgG anti-GQ1b antibodies

Table 2.
Summary of the clinical subtypes of Guillain-Barre syndrome.

Zika virus belongs to the virus family Flaviviridae. This virus was first isolated in 1947 from a monkey in the Zika forest of Uganda. Zika virus spread mainly by Aedes mosquitos as well as by intrauterine transmission, blood and sexual intercourse [20]. Most cases of Zika virus infection are associated with mild symptoms such as fever, headache, maculopapular skin rash, red eyes (conjunctivitis) and joint or muscle pain [21–23].

The outbreak of Zika virus infection in Brazil in 2015 has been associated with a more serious neurological complication such as Guillain-Barre syndrome [24]. This outbreak has been also resulted in increase in the incidence of babies with microcephaly [25, 26].

During Zika outbreak in Brazil, patients who developed Guillain-Barre syndrome secondary to Zika virus infection were found to have a higher level of anti-ganglioside antibodies of both IgM and IgG isotypes as compared to other patients with Zika infection in the absence of GBS [27].

Since Zika virus associated with serious devastating neurological complications such as Guillain-Barre syndrome and congenital anomalies in the newborn babies, several methods have been developed in order to detect the virus in early course of infection. Nonstructural protein 1 (NS1) is considered to be an essential biomarker for early detection and diagnosis of Zika virus. The development of double-antibody sandwich ELISA (DAS-ELISA) has been also used for early and rapid detection of ZIKA-NS1 protein in patients who newly infected with Zika virus [28].

At the present time, there is no antiviral treatment or specific vaccines approved for patients infected with Zika virus. Supportive care remains the main modality of managing these patients, yet the challenge remains to prevent congenital Zika syndrome in pregnant women [29].

4. Diagnosis of Guillain-Barre syndrome and Miller Fisher variant

The diagnosis of GBS and Miller Fisher variant is often made clinically based on the symptoms and clinical signs of the patients [30]. A more detail and supporting investigational studies such cerebrospinal fluid (CSF) analysis, electrophysiological tests such as nerve conduction studies, ultrasonographic and MRI imaging along with serologic testing can be carried out to confirm the diagnosis of GBS and other variants such as MFS [31].

Electrophysiological findings in patients with GBS suggestive of demyelination process in the form of reduce motor conduction velocity (MCV), prolonged motor distal latency and increase F wave latency. The findings of conduction block with absent H-reflex are considered to be the commonest and early sign in GBS [32].

Patients with Fisher-Bickerstaff syndrome (FBS) typically showed sensory axonal neuropathy in the form of reduced sensory nerve action potential (SNAP) amplitude in the absence of demyelination parameters [33].

The use of imaging studies such as peripheral nerve ultrasound and MRI are helpful diagnostic tools to diagnose inflammatory peripheral nerve roots [34].

The findings of MRI findings in patients with Miller-Fisher syndrome can range from cranial nerve involvement especially the optic nerve to severe cerebral white matter lesions [35, 36].

Another important biomarker which help confirming the diagnosis of GBS is the cerebrospinal fluid (CSF) analysis which typically show albuminocytologic dissociation (elevated protein level with normal cell count in cerebrospinal fluid) which has been also seen in patients with MFS and Bickerstaff brainstem encephalitis [37].

Although the diagnosis of MFS is based mainly on the classical trial of ophthalmoplegia, areflexia and ataxia which developed approximately within 1 week to 10 days after the initial infection, serologic tests can be used to confirm the diagnosis. The presence of anti-GQ1b antibodies, which was first described in 1992, provides a strong diagnostic marker for MFS [38].

The yield of this serological marker is high if the test done within 4 weeks after initial clinical onset [39].

5. Treatment practice of Guillain-Barre syndrome and Miller Fisher variant

Since GBS is a demyelinating polyneuropathy that cause rapid ascending muscle paralysis it is vitally important to admit patients with GBS to the intensive care unit for close monitoring and observation as over 30% of GBS patients can develop respiratory failure [40].

Currently plasmapheresis and intravenous immunoglobulin (IVIG) are the only effective therapies for GBS [41].

The timing of plasmapheresis has a significant impact on the clinical outcome if it is done within 2 weeks from the initial clinical onset as it reduces the time needed for ventilator support and improves motor function and walking without any help. The use of IVIG also shown to yield a good response in patients with GBS, however the use of plasmapheresis and IVIG were equally effective in GBS patients and combined therapy showed no significant difference in the final patients' clinical outcomes as compared to a single therapy. There is no role of corticosteroids therapy in the management of GBS even if it is used in high dose in the initial phase of GBS [40].

In patients with MFS IVIG have shown to speed the recovery of ophthalmoplegia and ataxia. However, IVIG and plasmapheresis have no significant impact on the overall outcome in patients with Miller Fisher syndrome [42].

6. Prognosis of Guillain-Barre syndrome and Miller Fisher variant

The overall prognosis of GBS is positive. Not all patients with GBS show complete recovery; however, most of these patients have a good outcome on one year follow up [43].

However, factors that indicate poor prognosis in GBS patients include old age and severe neurological deficit with cranial nerve injury at clinical onset, the need for mechanical ventilation and axonal damage in the nerve conduction study (**Table 3**) [44].

MFS has an overall a good prognosis [45], and despite the fact it has self-limiting course in most cases, Miller Fisher rarely progressive to respiratory failure [46].

The early diagnosis of MFS and early treatment with plasma exchange or intravenous immunoglobulins can reduce the severity of the disease and hasten the recovery in patients with MFS [46].

The ataxia and ophthalmoplegia usually recover within 1 to 3 months after initial clinical onset with almost complete resolution within 6 months. The loss of deep tendon reflexes may persist however does not interfere with daily functional activities [47].

1. Elderly patients
2. Severe focal neurological deficit at the initial presentation
3. Mechanical ventilation
4. Axonal demyelination in nerve conduction study

Table 3.
Poor prognostic factors in GBS [44].

7. Conclusion

Guillain-Barre syndrome is a serious neurological disorder associated with a rapid progressive ascending muscle paralysis. It is essential to provide maximum supportive medical care and start early therapy to prevent further deterioration and improve the future outcome of the patients.

Miller Fisher is a variant of Guillain-Barre syndrome is rare in pediatric population with an overall good prognosis. Early recognition and management of such uncommon neurological disorder will help in preventing further complications and long-term morbidity.

Conflict of interest

The author declares no conflict of interest.

Abbreviations

GBS	Guillain-Barre syndrome
MFS	Miller Fisher syndrome
PCB	pharyngeal-cervical brachial
MRI	magnetic resonance imaging
IVIG	intravenous immunoglobulin
ELISA	enzyme-linked immunosorbent assay

Author details

Raafat Hammad Seroor Jadah
Department of Pediatrics, Bahrain Defence Force Hospital, Royal Medical Services, Kingdom of Bahrain

*Address all correspondence to: nader212@hotmail.com

References

[1] Freitas MRG, Vidal CM, Orsini M. Guillain-Barre syndrome: Celebrating a century. Arquivos de Neuro-Psiquiatria. 2017;**75**(8):600-603. DOI: 10.1590/0004-282X20170093

[2] Leonhard SE, Mandarakas MR, Gondim FAA, Bateman K, Ferreira MLB, Cornblath DR. Diagnosis and management of Guillain-Barre syndrome in ten steps. Nature Reviews. Neurology. 2019;**15**(11):671-683. DOI: 10.1038/s41582-019-0250-9

[3] Willison HJ, Jacobs BC, Van Doorn PA. Guillain-Barre syndrome. Lancet. 2016;**388**(10045):717-727. DOI: 10.1016/S0140-6736(16)00339-1

[4] Estridge R, Iskander M. Understanding Guillain-Barre syndrome. JAAPA. 2015;**28**(7):19-22. DOI: 10.1097/01.JAA.000466585.10595.f5

[5] Ramirez-Zamora M, Burgos-Ganuza CR, Alas-Valle DA, Vergara-Galan PE, Ortez-Gonzalez CI. Guillain-Barre syndrome in pediatric age: Epidemiological, clinical and therapeutic profile in a hospital in El Salvador. Revista de Neurologia. 2009;**48**(6):292-296. DOI: 10.33588/rn.4806.2008560

[6] Ryan MM. Pediatric Guillain-Barre syndrome. Current Opinion in Pediatrics. 2013;**25**(6):689-693. DOI: 10.1097/MOP.0b013e328365ad3f

[7] Bandeira LP, Palaoro LG, Degenszajn J. Miller Fisher syndrome: A rare variant of Guillain-Barre syndrome. Autopsy & Case Reports. 2012;**2**(3):57-61. DOI: 10.4322/acr.2012.027

[8] Koike H. Zika virus and Guillain-Barre syndrome. Brain and Nerve. 2018;**70**(2):113-120. DOI: 10.11477/mf.1416200963

[9] Rodrigues-Morales AJ, Failoc-Rojas VE, Diaz-Velez C. Gastrointestinal, respiratory and/or arboviral infections? What is the cause of the Guillain-Barre syndrome epidemics in Peru? Current status—2019. Travel Medicine and Infectious Disease. 2019;**30**:114-116. DOI: 10.1016/j.tmaid.2019.06.015

[10] Rodriguez Y, Rojas M, Pacheco Y, Acosta-Ampudia Y, Ramirez-Santana C, Monsalve DM, et al. Guillain-Barré syndrome, transverse myelitis and infectious disease. Cellular & Molecular Immunology. 2018;**15**(6):547-562. DOI: 10.1038/cmi.2017.142

[11] Liu S, Dong C, Ubogu EE. Immunotherapy of Guillain-Barre syndrome. Human Vaccines & Immunotherapeutics. 2018;**14**(11):2568-2579. DOI: 10.1080/21645515.2018.1493415

[12] Dagklis IE, Papaglannopoulos S, Theodoridou V, Kazis D, Argyopoulou O, Bostantjopoulou S. Miller-Fisher syndrome: Are anti-GAD antibodies implicated in its pathophysiology? Case Reports in Neurological Medicine. 2016;**2016**:3431849. DOI: 10.1155/2016/3431849

[13] Kilic B, Gungor S, Ozgor B. Clinical, electrophysiological findings and evaluation of prognosis of patients with Guillain-Barre syndrome. The Turkish Journal of Pediatrics. 2019;**61**(2):200-208. DOI: 10.24953/turkjped.2019.02.008

[14] Walling AD, Dickson G. Guillain-Barre syndrome. American Family Physician. 2013;**87**(3):191-197. Available from: https://www.ncbi.nlm.nih.gov/pubmed/23418763

[15] Liu DY, Hollenbacj JR, Gregorin JA, Wynbrandt JH. A case of acute motor sensory axonal neuropathy: A variant of Gillian-Barre syndrome, with possible syndrome of irreversible

lithium-effectuated neurotoxicity. Case Reports in Medicine. 2020;**2020**:4683507. DOI: 10.1155/2020/4683507

[16] Pradhan RR, Yadav SK, Yadav SK Sr. Pharyngeal-cervical-branchial variant of Guillain-Barre syndrome in children. Cureus. 2020 Feb;**12**(2):e6983. DOI: 10.7759/cureus.6983

[17] Wakerley BR, Yuki N. Pharyngeal-cervical-branchial variant of Guillain-Barre syndrome. Journal of Neurology, Neurosurgery, and Psychiatry. 2014;**85**(3):339-344. DOI: 10.1136/jnnp-2013-305397

[18] Aranyi Z, Kovacs T, Sipos I, Bereczki D. Miller Fisher syndrome: Brief overview and update with a focus on electrophysiological findings. European Journal of Neurology. 2012;**19**(1):15-20. DOI: 10.1111/j.1468-1331.2011.03445.x

[19] Kuwabara S. Fisher syndrome and Bickerstaff brainstem encephalitis. Brain and Nerve. 2015;**67**(11):1371-1376. DOI: 10.11477/mf.1416200308

[20] Karam E, Giraldo J, Rodrigues F, Hernandez-Pereira CE, Rodrigues-Morales AJ, Blohm GM, et al. Ocular flutter following zika virus infection. Journal of Neurovirology. 2017;**23**(6):932-934. DOI: 10.1007/s13365-017-0585-1

[21] Wikan N, Smith DR. Zika virus: History of a newly emerging arbovirus. The Lancet Infectious Diseases. 2016;**16**(7):e119-e126. DOI: 10.1016/S1473-3099(16)30010-X

[22] Guillier A, Amazan E, Aoun A, Baubion E, Derancourt C. Zika virus infection: A review. Annales de Dermatologie et de Vénéréologie. 2017;**144**(8-9):518-524. DOI: 10.1016/j.annder.2017.05.013

[23] Zombrano LI, Fuentes-Barahona IC, Soto-Fernandez RJ, Zuniga C, de Silva JC, Rodrigues-Morales AJ. Guillain-Barre syndrome associated with zika virus infection in Honduras, 2016-2017. International Journal of Infectious Diseases. 2019;**84**:136-137. DOI: 10.1016/j.ijid.2019.05.008

[24] Koppolu V, Shantha RT. Zika virus outbreak: A review of neurological complications, diagnosis, and treatment options. Journal of Neurovirology. 2018;**24**(3):255-272. DOI: 10.1007/s13365-018-0614-8

[25] Pastrana A, Albarracin M, Hoffmann M, Delturco G, Lopez R, Gil R, et al. Congenital zika syndrome in Argentina: Case series study. Archivos Argentinos de Pediatría. 2019;**117**(6):e635-e639. DOI: 10.5546/aap.2019.e635

[26] Villamil-Gomez WE, Sanchez-Herrera AR, Hernandez H, Hernandez-Iriarte J, Diaz-Ricardo K, Castellanos J, et al. Guillain-Barre syndrome during the zika virus outbreak in Sucre, Columbia, 2016. Travel Medicine and Infectious Disease. 2017;**16**:62-63. DOI: 10.1016/j.tmaid-2017.03.012

[27] Rivera-Correa J, de Siqueira IC, Mota S, do Rosario MS, Pereira de Jesus PA, LCJ A, et al. Anti-ganglioside antibodies in patients with zika virus infection-associated Guillain-Barre syndrome in Brazil. PLoS Neglected Tropical Diseases. 2019;**13**(9):e0007695. DOI: 10.1371/journal.pntd.0007695

[28] Zhang L, Du X, Chen C, Chen Z, Zhang L, Han Q, et al. Development and characterization of double-antibody sandwich ELISA for detection of Zika virus infection. Viruses. 2018;**10**(11):634. DOI: 10.3390/v10110634

[29] Ferraris P, Yssel H, Misse D. Zika virus infection: An update. Microbes and Infection. 2019;**21**(8-9):353-360. DOI: 10.1016/j.micinf.2019.04.005

[30] Villamil-Gomez W, Silvera LA, Paez-Castellanos J, Rodriguez-Morales AJ. Guillain-Barre syndrome after Chikungunya infection: A case in Columbia. Enfermedades Infecciosas y Microbiología Clínica. 2016;**34**(2):140-141. DOI: 10.1016/j.eimc.2015.05.012

[31] Al Othman B, Raabe J, Kini A, Lee AG. Update: The Miller Fisher variants of Guillain-Barre syndrome. Current Opinion in Ophthalmology. 2019;**30**(6):462-466. DOI: 10.1097/ICU.0000000000000611

[32] Sudulgunta SR, Sodalgunta MB, Sepehrar M, Khorram H, Bangalore Raja SK, Kothandapani S, et al. Guillain-Barre syndrome: Clinical profile and management. German Medical Science. 2015;**13**(16):1-15. DOI: 10.3205/000220. eCollection 2015

[33] Alberti MA, Povedano M, Montero J, Casasnovas C. Early electrophysiological findings in Fisher-Bickerstaff syndrome. Neurología. 2017. pii:S0213-4853(17)30241-4. DOI: 10.1016/j.nrl.2017.05.012

[34] Doets AY, Jacobs BC, Van Doorn PA. Advances in management of Guillain-Barre syndrome. Current Opinion in Neurology. 2018;**31**(5):541-550. DOI: 10.1097/WCO.0000000000000602

[35] Malhotra A, Zhang M, Wu X, Jindal S, Durand D, Makhani N. MRI findings of optic pathway involvement in Miller Fisher syndrome in 3 pediatric patients and a review of the literature. Journal of Clinical Neuroscience. 2017;**39**:63-67. DOI: 10.1016/j.jocn.2016.12.049

[36] Xu Y, Liu L. Miller-Fisher syndrome associated with unilateral cerebral white matter lesions. Neurologia i Neurochirurgia Polska. 2015;**49**(5):344-347. DOI: 10.1016/j.pjnns.2015.07.008

[37] Illes Z, Blaabjerg M. Cerebrospinal fluid findings in Guillain-Barre syndrome and chronic inflammatory demyelinating polyneuropathies. Handbook of Clinical Neurology. 2017;**146**:125-138. DOI: 10.1016/B978-0-12-804279-3.00009-5

[38] Yepishin IV, Allison RZ, Kaminskas DA, Zagorski NM, Liow KK. Miller Fisher syndrome: A case report highlighting heterogeneity of clinical features and focused differential diagnosis. Hawaii Journal of Medicine & Public Health. 2016;**75**(7):196-199. Available from: https://www.ncbi.nlm.nih.gov/pubmed/27437164

[39] Rojas-Garcia R, Gallardo E, Serrano-Munuera C, de Luna N, Ortiz E, Roig C, et al. Anti-GQ1b antibodies: Usefulness of its detection for the diagnosis of Miller-Fisher syndrome. Medicina Clínica (Barcelona). 2001;**116**(20):761-764. DOI: 10.1016/s0025-7753(01)71980-x

[40] Dimachkie MM, Barohn RJ. Guillain-Barre syndrome and variants. Neurologic Clinics. 2013;**31**(2):491-510. DOI: 10.1016/j.ncl.2013.01.005

[41] Verboon C, Doets AY, Galassi G, Davidson A, Waheed W, Pereon Y, et al. Current treatment practice of Guillain-Barre syndrome. Neurology. 2019;**93**(1):e59-e76. DOI: 10.1212/WNL.0000000000007719

[42] Van Doorn PA. Diagnosis, treatment and prognosis of Guillain-Barre syndrome (GBS). Presse Médicale. 2013;**42**(6 Pt 2):e193-e201. DOI: 10.1016/j.lpm.2013.02.328

[43] Wang Y, Lang W, Zhang Y, Ma X, Zhou C, Zhang HL. Long-term prognosis of Guillain-Barre syndrome not determined by treatment options? Oncotarget. 2017;**8**(45):79991-80001. DOI: 10.18632/oncotarget.20620

[44] Gonzalez-Suarez I, Sanz-Gallego I, Rodriguez de Rivera FJ, Arpa J. Guillain-Barre syndrome: Natural history

and prognostic factors: A retrospective review of 106 cases. BMC Neurology. 2013;**13**:95. DOI: 10.1186/1471-2377-13-95

[45] Teener JW. Miller Fisher's syndrome. Seminars in Neurology. 2012;**32**(5):512-516. DOI: 10.1055/s-0033-1334470

[46] Mwansa H, Obiekezie O, Kaneria S. A case of Miller Fisher syndrome. The American Journal of Medicine. 2019;**132**(6):e591-e592. DOI: 10.1016/j.amjmed.2019.01.014

[47] Bukhari S, Taboada J. A case of Miller Fisher syndrome and literature review. Cureus. 2017;**9**(2):e1048. DOI: 10.7759/cureus.1048

Chapter 7

Neuromuscular Effects and Rehabilitation in Guillain-Barré Syndrome Associated with Zika Virus Infection

Thomas Harbo and Henning Andersen

Abstract

The 2015–2017 Zika Virus outbreak caused a high increase in patients with Guillain-Barré syndrome (GBS), a post infectious autoimmune disease of the peripheral nerves. The severity of GBS can range from mild impairment with fast recovery to complete paralysis including severe respiratory or autonomic failure. Recovery may take months and even years and may be incomplete despite disease modifying treatment with IVIG or plasma exchange. Therefore, optimal supportive care and effective rehabilitation remain crucial. Multidisciplinary rehabilitation is recommended but may be challenging in the acute phase because of limited patient participation due to profound muscle weakness and severe pain. Inactive denervated muscles will inevitably undergo rapid degeneration resulting in wasting, weakness, and contractures as major long-term complications in severely affected patients. In this chapter, the current evidence of rehabilitation on the short- and long-term motor function in GBS is reviewed, including newly obtained experiences with neuromuscular electrical stimulation (NMES). Rehabilitation remains an area lacking well designed and controlled clinical studies and thus a clear lack of evidence-based guidelines.

Keywords: Guillain Barré syndrome, prognosis, chronic disability, rehabilitation, exercise, neuromuscular electrical stimulation

1. Introduction

Guillain Barré Syndrome (GBS) is an acute inflammatory disease affecting peripheral nerves and nerve roots [1, 2]. Most commonly, GBS is preceded by an infection a few weeks prior to neuropathic symptoms [3]. Thus, incidence of GBS can increase during outbreaks of infectious diseases. This was most recently observed during the 2015 to 2017 Zika Virus epidemic in the French Polynesia and Latin America with a highly increased incidence of GBS in several countries [4–9]. GBS typically presents with muscle weakness and sensory symptoms combined with loss of tendon reflexes. Symptoms initially present in the lower extremities progressing to the upper extremities and the respiratory and cranial muscles [10]. The progressive phase usually last for days to weeks with most patients reaching nadir within four weeks of symptom debut followed by a plateau phase and a slow

IntechOpen

recovery. Beside the typical presentation of sensory and motor neuropathy, patients may have clinical variants like the triad of ophthalmoplegia, ataxia and areflexia known as the Miller Fischer Syndrome, pure motor, paraparetic or pharyngea-cervical-brachial variant [11], and in association with Zika Virus infection a case of GBS with ocular flutter, ataxia, tetraparesis and areflexia has been reported [12]. Furthermore, neuropathy can be classified as demyelinating or axonal according to the electrophysiological examination [13].

The prognosis of GBS is very heterogeneous. Some patients are mildly affected with a fast recovery and no disabilities irrespective of receiving any treatment. Between 20 and 30% of patients develop complete paralysis, severe respiratory or autonomic failure and receive treatment in the intensive care unit (ICU) for months [14]. In a group of prolonged mechanically ventilated patients, 31% were able to walk after one year and 58% after maximum time of follow up [15]. The sudden increase of patients with Zika Virus-related GBS was a challenge for health care systems in low income countries such as Brazil with limited resources for diagnostics, treatment, ICU capacity as well as rehabilitation facilities [1, 2]. Despite the lack of evidence, multidisciplinary supportive care and rehabilitation are important in GBS. In the acute phase, consensus- based recommendations include (1) monitoring of respiratory and autonomic function in a setting with available artificial ventilation and neuro-intensive care, (2) prophylactic antithrombotic treatment for deep vein thrombosis, (3) pain management, (4) management of nutrition as well as bladder and bowel dysfunction and (5) physiotherapy to prevent muscle shortening and joint contractures [16]. All of these interventions should be followed by a rehabilitation and exercise program to regain physical abilities as fast as possible. Recovery can take months and even years and end up with significant chronic disabilities despite immunomodulatory treatment. As shown in the largest prospective cohort of patients with GBS studied to date, a large proportion of patients had long-term motor dysfunction with 17% of patients from Europe and America were unable to walk unaided after 12 months [17], emphasizing the importance of identifying more effective neuromuscular rehabilitation. Motor dysfunctions such as weakness, wasting and contractures are major long-term complications in severely affected patients. In this review, we present an overview of existing evidence of treatment to prevent muscle weakness and disabilities after GBS with special emphasis on the effect of neuromuscular rehabilitation in the acute and chronic phases of the disease.

2. Treatment and rehabilitation in GBS

Pharmacological treatment. In several large randomized controlled clinical trials, treatment with plasma exchange (PE) or intravenous immunoglobulin (IVIG) initiated in the acute phase of GBS have proven effective. Compared to placebo, treatment with PE or IVIG result in reduced need for respiratory support and an increased chance to regain mobility and muscle strength after 1 month and 12 months [18, 19]. Despite immunomodulatory treatment, a group of patients with GBS still have a very poor prognosis. In a combined cohort study of 526 patients and a cross sectional study including 63 ventilated patients [15], 6% of patients with GBS required mechanical ventilation for more than two months. The prolonged mechanically ventilated patients had a median (range) length of stay at the ICU of 101 (97–126) days and at hospital of 129 (104–162) days, followed by 252 (177–403) days of clinical rehabilitation and 198 (183–502) days of outpatient rehabilitation. At 11 years follow-up, only 58% had regained ambulation and the median time to regain ambulation was

548 (270–730) days. This emphasizes the need for more effective treatment in GBS. Recently, small clinical studies have indicated that monoclonal antibodies against complement proteins given in the early phase of the disease could have some benefit in GBS; however, larger studies are needed to confirm this [20, 21]. It is important to underline that there are currently no evidence-based pharmacological treatments available to prevent muscle atrophy or muscle weakness in GBS [22].

Multidisciplinary rehabilitation. Most patients with moderate to severe GBS are offered multidisciplinary rehabilitation, which means two or more coordinated interventions under medical supervision by a neurologist or rehabilitation physician. Multidisciplinary rehabilitation aims at regaining autonomy with the ability to perform all activities of daily living. This may include physiotherapy or occupational therapy and exercise programs, but also nursing, dietary advice, psychotherapy, speech therapy, and social rehabilitation depending on the needs of the individual patient. The individualized approach to multidisciplinary rehabilitation as well as a considerably variability in facilities between countries and hospitals compromise the possibility to design research trials to assess the efficacy of a multidisciplinary rehabilitation intervention. In a systematic review of rehabilitation interventions in patients with GBS [23], only five original studies could be identified evaluating the effectiveness of multidisciplinary rehabilitation. These studies include only one good quality randomized controlled study comparing high and low intensity rehabilitation in patients with remaining disability more than one year after GBS [24]. In this study, 79 adult patients were included 1–12 years after the GBS diagnosis and randomized to receive either individualized outpatient-based high-intensive rehabilitation (intervention, n = 40) or a lower intensity home-based program (control, n = 39). The intervention comprised three one-hour individualized sessions weekly for 12 weeks. Sessions included physical and occupational therapy for strengthening, endurance and gait training as well as specific rehabilitation tasks to improve everyday life activities as well as community and work functions. The control group completed a 30-minute maintenance training program twice weekly and was also allowed to perform other rehabilitation activities if needed. Outcome was assessed one year after the intervention and included measurements of activity level, participation, and perceived impact of disease-related problems. Based on the total and the motor scales of the Functional Independence Measure (FIM) in an intention to treat analysis, there was a small but statistically significant improvement in the high intensity rehabilitation group compared to the controls. Furthermore, 80% of the patients complying with the high intensity protocol had a clinically meaningful improvement in the FIM motor score (at least 3 points) compared with only 8% of controls. Adverse effects were not reported; however, only 22 (55%) of the 40 patients assigned to high intensity rehabilitation completed the study due to loss to follow up or inability or unwillingness to comply with the protocol. This low number of follow-up reduces the applicability and external validity of the study suggesting that applicability of the intervention is challenging. Other original studies have included: (1) one case control study (n = 34) of inpatient rehabilitation with a control group of healthy subjects [25], (2) one prospective case series (n = 35) of inpatient rehabilitation followed by a home-based training program [26], and (3) two retrospective case series (n = 39 and 24) of inpatient rehabilitation [27, 28]. In these studies, patients with GBS improved during multidisciplinary rehabilitation but the studies were not designed to distinguish between spontaneous recovery and the effect of the rehabilitation intervention.

Despite several limitations, the authors of the review concluded that there is good evidence (Grade level II) to support ambulatory, outpatient multidisciplinary rehabilitation to obtain long-term improvements in levels of activity and participation in patients with GBS in the later stages of recovery. Further, the authors concluded that there is satisfactory (Grade level III) evidence to support (1) inpatient rehabilitation followed by outpatient rehabilitation thereby inducing functional recovery and (2) physical therapy and exercise to reduce joint contractures and muscle weakness. In another more recent case series of 51 patients with GBS, motor recovery following the acute pharmacological treatment response was assessed during the acute inpatient care as well as after outpatient and homebased rehabilitation [29]. A description of the intervention was not provided, but it included physical therapy for 61 ± 58 (mean ± SD) days for inpatients, 96 ± 70 days for outpatients, and 75 ± 15 days during home rehabilitation. Again, the natural history with spontaneous improvement after GBS and the lack of a control group impairs the possibility to draw any final conclusions based on this study regarding the effectiveness of rehabilitation. However, it was shown that muscle strength measured with a MRC sum score [30] and ambulation assessed with the GBS disability score [31] continue to improve beyond the first six months of rehabilitation.

Exercise. In a systematic review, Simatos and colleagues evaluated the available literature on exercise as an intervention in the rehabilitation of adult patients with GBS [32]. Studies between 1951 and 2016 were identified in PubMed searches and the quality of the studies was assessed and classified according to a modified version of the Centre for Evidence-Based Medicine level of evidence. Seven studies with exercise as the main intervention were identified, including four uncontrolled single cases with a low evidence level, one trial including multidisciplinary rehabilitation (reviewed in the previous section), [24], and two Dutch studies of a case series in an open label standardized exercise protocol (evidence level 5) [33, 34]. In the Dutch study, 16 patients were included between six months and 15 years after their GBS diagnosis as well as four patients with stable chronic inflammatory demyelinating polyradiculoneuropathy. All patients were ambulatory and reported fatigue as a major complaint. The exercise intervention consisted of three 45-minute bicycling sessions every week for 12 weeks. During the 12-week period, training intensity was gradually increased. The target heart rate increasing from 65% to a maximum of 90% of maximal heart rate and an increasing workload was applied on the bicycle home trainer. The intervention resulted in lower fatigue levels, increased isokinetic muscle strength and a higher peak oxygen uptake. Further, patients improved on a handicap scale and on the physical components score of the SF36 Quality of Life scale. Two patients did not complete the study for non-study related reasons, and 25% reported mild and transient muscle cramps, paresthesia, or pain. Overall, exercise as an intervention in patients with late disabilities and fatigue in GBS is feasible and may benefit some patients.

Neuromuscular electrical stimulation (NMES). In the acute phase of severe GBS, rehabilitation exercise is challenged by limited patient participation due to severe weakness or even paralysis. For practical reasons, exercise may also be challenged if patients are in the ICU, intubated and on ventilator support. Inactive and denervated muscles will indisputably and fast degenerate and muscle atrophy will develop [35, 36]. NMES is a method to induce muscle contractions without patient participation. This may be an alternative therapeutic approach in the acute phase of GBS, which can minimize inactivation and denervation wasting until patients have recovered to a level where a multidisciplinary rehabilitation effort can be initiated [37, 38]. In a small proof of concept study this has proven feasible with satisfactory safety. There was also a trend for an effect of

NMES on muscle wasting as an add on to established standard of care in the acute and subacute phases of GBS [39]. Seventeen patients with moderate to severe GBS were randomized to receive an hour of NMES on weekdays on the right or left quadriceps femoral muscle with the non-stimulated muscle serving as control. Stimulation was initiated within two weeks after the first sign of weakness and was continued through the acute hospital admission and the following inpatient rehabilitation. The median (range) time of participation was 27 days (10–95) and included 17 (4–53) stimulation sessions. During the study, each patient had a mean loss of lean body mass (muscle) of 3.4 kg, establishing that patients with GBS will experience substantial muscle wasting. NMES was found to be safe and feasible as an add on to standard supportive therapy and rehabilitation in the acute and subacute phases of GBS. There was a trend towards a preventive effect of NMES on muscle atrophy, but the study was not designed to explore effect on patient disability.

Virtual Motor Rehabilitation System. Virtual Motor Rehabilitation (VMR) is a new technology combining novel rehabilitation software with low cost commercially available devices such as the Nintendo® Wii platform. To be effective, multidisciplinary rehabilitation in GBS is very time demanding including several daily sessions for as long as 6, 12 and 18 months [40]. Often the rehabilitation offered is limited due to lack of time and resources, and patients may find training tedious and monotonous, resulting in lack of compliance. Therefore, VMR could be an attractive supplement to the established rehabilitation regimen. The method is still under development and so far only one study has been published, describing VMR applied four and five months after admission in two patients with severe GBS as an add on to the conventional multidisciplinary rehabilitation [41]. In this study, the Nintendo® Wii Balance Board and a virtual environmental tool were applied in 20 rehabilitation sessions consisting of 30 minutes of traditional therapy and 30 minutes of VMR. Compliance was good and patients' status improved. VMR could be developed further to include more aspects of the rehabilitation process in the future.

Safety. In anecdotal case reports and experimental animal studies it has been indicated that over-exercising during rehabilitation after GBS may damage motor units and cause paradoxical weakening, which has led to hesitation concerning the recommendation to do intensive and strenuous exercise [16]. The clinical data to support this concern are negligible and overall, it is reasonable to believe that the benefit of exercising weakened muscles after GBS excess the risk of harm. However, systematic registration of safety and complications should always be included in future studies.

3. Conclusions

Neuromuscular rehabilitation after GBS is important for the functional outcome of each individual patient. Studied rehabilitation interventions in the acute, subacute/intermediate, and chronic/long-term phase are summarized in **Figure 1**. However, the quality of the present evidence of rehabilitation efficacy is low, rehabilitation is both complex, time consuming and expensive, and there is currently no standardized care for patients with neuromuscular disabilities after GBS. Therefore, the rehabilitation effort may lack necessary resources and expertise. Because the monophasic course and spontaneous recovery in GBS challenge the interpretation of non-controlled studies, future large controlled studies and standardized sensitive efficacy outcome measures are needed to improve the interpretation of neuromuscular rehabilitation trials in GBS.

Acute phase (1-8 weeks) **Patients are at risk of deteriorating and to suffer complications**	Rehabilitation focus (no grade 1 or 2 evidence)
Patients are at hospital for acute care including respiratory and autonomic monitoring and support, thromboprophylaxis, pain treatment etc.	* Physiotherapy to prevent muscle shortening and contractures. * Neuromuscular electrical stimulation. Safe and feasible, efficacy still to be explored.
Intermediate phase (weeks to several months) **Patients improve gradually**	Rehabilitation focus: Regain autonomy and ability to perform activities of daily living. (no grade 1 or 2 evidence)
Patients are at rehabilitation centers or outpatient rehabilitation facilities.	* Multidisciplinary rehabilitation * Task specific training * Neuromuscular electrical stimulation. Safe and feasible, efficacy still to be determined. * Cardiovascular and strengthening exercises
Chronic phase (months to years) **Patients are stable with residual disabilities**	Rehabilitation focus: Further improve or maintain function
Patients are exercising and performing rehabilitation training at home, at outpatient facilities or fitness centers.	* High intensity multidisciplinary rehabilitation improves functional independence **(grade level 2)**. * Multidisciplinary rehabilitation * Task specific training * Exercise cardiovascular and strength * Virtual Motor Rehabilitation

Figure 1.
Neuromuscular rehabilitation in three phases of Guillain Barré syndrome. Rehabilitation focus and studied interventions in three phases of Guillain Barré syndrome, the acute, subacute/intermediate, and chronic/ long-term phase. Level of evidence is indicated using the following grade system: Level 1, meta-analysis of multiple well designed randomized controlled trials; level 2, at least one randomized controlled trial; level 3–5, non-randomized controlled trials, descriptive studies or case series.

4. Policy and procedures

Neuromuscular Electrical Stimulation Protocol.

Stimulation of the quadriceps muscle was performed using a STIWELL med4 stimulation unit, https://www.ottobock.co.th/neurorehabilitation/solutions/solutions-with-functional-electrical-stimulation/stiwell-med-4/(Otto Bock, Konigsee, Germany) and two large stimulation pads (6 × 8 cm). The intensity of electrical stimulation was titrated individually at entry and weekly during the study to the point of maximal contraction or the highest tolerable intensity. During the first session of stimulation, the skin under the pads was inspected every five minutes for redness or other signs of tissue damage. Trained physical therapists attached the equipment and titrated the stimulation intensity, but after being attached to the patient the individualized stimulation protocol ran automatically.

Direct muscle fiber stimulation (MFS). With MFS, contraction is induced directly through the muscle fiber membrane independent of the neuromuscular junction, which means that complete distally denervated muscle fibers can be activated. The disadvantage is that higher intensity stimulation, especially in atrophic muscle, is needed which may cause discomfort and skin irritation. MFS was applied by placing two pads over the proximal and distal part of the muscle (**Figure 2**) with triangular dual-phase stimulation pulses. The initiation protocol was 1 Hz frequency,

DOI: http://dx.doi.org/10.5772/intechopen.93930

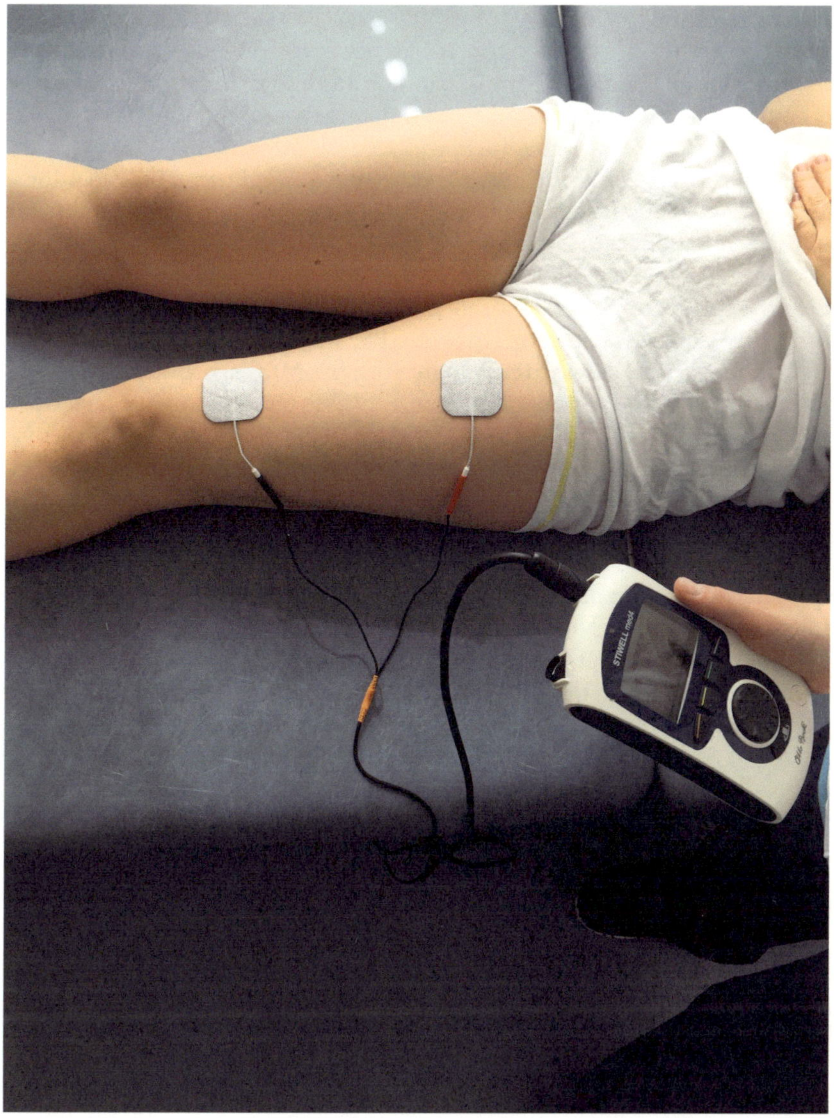

Figure 2.
Electrical muscle stimulation. A healthy control subject with electrodes in place for direct muscle fiber stimulation of the left quadriceps femoris muscle by the STIWELL med4 stimulation unit.

250 ms pulse width, and 3/6 on/off ratio. The lowest pulse width with maximal contraction was chosen and frequency was increased to the highest tolerated level.

Neuromuscular electrical stimulation (NMES). With NMES the muscle is activated through the muscle spindle and neuromuscular endplate. As a result, the contraction is more physiological and less electrical stimulation is needed. NMES was applied by one pad placed on the middle of the muscle bulk, where the neuromuscular transmission is located with rectangular dual-phase stimulation pulses. The protocol included four phases of 5, 15, 15, and 5 minutes, with frequencies of 10, 40, 60, 3 Hz, with a pulse width of 0.3 ms. Intensity could be adjusted from 0 to 100 mA and was increased to the highest tolerated level.

The intention was to stimulate patients five to seven days a week including 20 minutes of MFS followed by 40 minutes of NMES. Also, the NMES was applied to patients where no visible contraction could be observed.

5. Mini-dictionary of terms

Neuromuscular Electrical Stimulation: A method to induce muscle contraction by applying an electrical impulse to the neuromuscular endplate by an electronic device.

Multidisciplinary rehabilitation: Two or more coordinated interventions for disabled patients to regain autonomy and functions of daily living. Usually, multidisciplinary rehabilitation is performed by physical therapists and occupational therapists but may include other professions.

Motor dysfunction: Several methods are used to describe motor dysfunction in GBS. Muscle weakness is a main feature of GBS, which develops quickly in the acute phase. Weakness can be assessed manually with the MRC score on a scale from 0 to 5. (0, paralysis with no visible contraction; 1, visible contraction but no limb movement; 2, limb movement only with gravity eliminated; 3, active movement against gravity; 4, active movement against gravity and resistance but reduced strength; 5, normal strength). Weakness may be quantified on a linear scale using a dynamometer [42]. In addition to weakness, chronic muscle dysfunction can result in muscle wasting, and muscle and joint contractures and shortening, which is very disabling.

Impairment and disability: Impairment is the direct damage caused by the disease, for example weakness of leg muscles (as described above) or loss of sensation, while disability is the loss of the function caused by the impairment, for example loss of ambulation. Often, the GBS disability score is used to describe the severity of the disease concerning the level of disability. (0, healthy; 1, minor symptoms and capable of running; 2, able to walk 10 m without assistance but unable to run; 3, able to walk 10 m across an open space with help; 4 bedridden or chair bound; 4, requiring assisted ventilation for at least part of the day; 6, death).

6. Key facts of neuromuscular rehabilitation in GBS

Neuromuscular rehabilitation in Guillain Barré Syndrome can include

- Physical therapy to prevent muscle and joint shortening and contractures.
- Multidisciplinary rehabilitation with two or more coordinated interventions for disabled patients to regain autonomy and functions of daily living.
- Exercise and training to improve or maintain physical functioning.
- Neuromuscular electrical stimulation to prevent muscle wasting.

The prognosis of Guillain Barré Syndrome

- Guillain Barré Syndrome is a heterogenous disorder with a monophasic course.
- Clinical severity ranges from mild impairment to complete paralysis combined with respiratory and autonomic failure.
- In 20 to 30% of patients, mechanical ventilation is required at nadir of GBS.
- The most severely affected patients have a long recovery phase and a poor prognosis.
- More than half of all mechanically ventilated patients are unable to walk unassisted at one year follow up.

7. Summary points of neuromuscular rehabilitation in GBS

- Most commonly, GBS is preceded by an infection, therefore, the incidence of GBS can increase during outbreaks of infectious diseases, which was most recently observed during the Zika Virus outbreak in the French Polynesia and Latin America with a high increase in the incidence of GBS in several countries.

- Despite optimal evidence-based treatment with immunoglobulin and plasma exchange, a large proportion of patients with GBS will have substantial neuromuscular disabilities more than one year after disease onset. Among patients receiving mechanical ventilation, more than half will be able to walk unassisted.

- In the acute phase of GBS, physical therapy is important to prevent muscle shortening and joint contractures.

- Patients may still improve their physical function several years after onset of GBS.

- There is evidence to support high intensity multidisciplinary rehabilitation and exercise which improves level of activity and participation in the late and chronic stages of GBS.

- New approaches like Neuromuscular Electrical Stimulation and Virtual Motor Rehabilitation seem to be feasible methods in the acute and late stage recovery of GBS, but efficacy needs to be explored in future studies.

Abbreviations

FIM	functional independence measure
GBS	Guillain Barré syndrome
ICU	intensive care unit
IVIG	intravenous immunoglobulin
MFS	muscle fiber stimulation
NMES	neuromuscular electrical stimulation
PE	plasma exchange
VMR	virtual motor rehabilitation

Author details

Thomas Harbo* and Henning Andersen
Department of Neurology, Aarhus University Hospital, Aarhus, Denmark

*Address all correspondence to: tharbo@dadlnet.dk

References

[1] Leonhard SE, Conde RM, de Assis Aquino GF, Jacobs BC. Diagnosis and treatment of Guillain-Barre syndrome during the Zika virus epidemic in Brazil: A national survey study. J.Peripher.Nerv. Syst. 2019a;**24**(4):340-347 available from: PM:31746070

[2] Leonhard SE, Mandarakas MR, Gondim FAA, Bateman K, Ferreira MLB, Cornblath DR, et al. Diagnosis and management of Guillain-Barre syndrome in ten steps. Nat.Rev.Neurol. 2019b;**15**(11):671-683 available from: PM:31541214

[3] Sipila JO, Soilu-Hanninen M. The incidence and triggers of adult-onset Guillain-Barre syndrome in southwestern Finland 2004-2013. European Journal of Neurology. 2015;**22**(2):292-298 available from: PM:25196425

[4] Cao-Lormeau VM, Blake A, Mons S, Lastere S, Roche C, Vanhomwegen J, et al. Guillain-Barre syndrome outbreak associated with Zika virus infection in French Polynesia: A case-control study. Lancet. 2016;**387**(10027):1531-1539 available from: PM:26948433

[5] Cardona-Ospina, J.A., Henao-SanMartin, V., Acevedo-Mendoza, W.F., Nasner-Posso, K.M., Martinez-Pulgarin, D.F., Restrepo-Lopez, A., Valencia-Gallego, V., Collins, M.H., & Rodriguez-Morales, A.J. 2019. Fatal Zika virus infection in the Americas: A systematic review. Int.J.Infect.Dis., 88, 49-59 available from: PM:31499212

[6] Parra, B., Lizarazo, J., Jimenez-Arango, J.A., Zea-Vera, A.F., Gonzalez-Manrique, G., Vargas, J., Angarita, J.A., Zuniga, G., Lopez-Gonzalez, R., Beltran, C.L., Rizcala, K.H., Morales, M.T., Pacheco, O., Ospina, M.L., Kumar, A., Cornblath, D.R., Munoz, L.S., Osorio, L., Barreras, P., & Pardo, C.A. 2016. Guillain-Barre syndrome associated with Zika virus infection in Colombia. *N.Engl.J.Med.*, 375, (16) 1513-1523 available from: PM:27705091

[7] Rodriguez-Morales AJ, Failoc-Rojas VE, Diaz-Velez C. Gastrointestinal, respiratory and/or arboviral infections? What is the cause of the Guillain-Barre syndrome epidemics in Peru? Current status - 2019. Travel.Med.Infect.Dis. 2019;**30**:114-116 available from: PM:31265907

[8] Villamil-Gomez WE, Sanchez-Herrera AR, Hernandez H, Hernandez-Iriarte J, Diaz-Ricardo K, Castellanos J, et al. Guillain-Barre syndrome during the Zika virus outbreak in Sucre, Colombia, 2016. Travel.Med.Infect.Dis. 2017;**16**:62-63 available from: PM:28347781

[9] Zambrano LI, Fuentes-Barahona IC, Soto-Fernandez RJ, Zuniga C, da Silva JC, Rodriguez-Morales AJ. Guillain-Barre syndrome associated with Zika virus infection in Honduras, 2016-2017. Int.J.Infect.Dis. 2019;**84**:136-137 available from: PM:31096053

[10] Willison HJ, Jacobs BC, van Doorn PA. Guillain-Barre syndrome. Lancet. 2016;**388**(10045):717-727 available from: PM:26948435

[11] Wakerley BR, Yuki N. Mimics and chameleons in Guillain-Barre and Miller fisher syndromes. Pract.Neurol. 2015;**15**(2):90-99 available from: PM:25239628

[12] Karam E, Giraldo J, Rodriguez F, Hernandez-Pereira CE, Rodriguez-Morales AJ, Blohm GM, et al. Ocular flutter following Zika virus infection. Journal of Neurovirology. 2017;**23**(6):932-934 available from: PM:29147884

[13] Hadden RD, Cornblath DR, Hughes RA, Zielasek J, Hartung HP,

Toyka KV, et al. Electrophysiological classification of Guillain-Barre syndrome: Clinical associations and outcome. Plasma exchange/ Sandoglobulin Guillain-Barre syndrome trial group. Annals of Neurology. 1998;**44**(5):780-788 available from: PM:9818934

[14] Al-Hakem H, Sindrup SH, Andersen H, de la Cour CD, Lassen LL, van den Berg B, et al. Guillain-Barre syndrome in Denmark: A population-based study on epidemiology, diagnosis and clinical severity. J.Neurol. 2019;**266**(2):440-449 available from: PM:30536111

[15] van den Berg B, Storm EF, Garssen MJP, Blomkwist-Markens PH, Jacobs BC. Clinical outcome of Guillain-Barre syndrome after prolonged mechanical ventilation. Journal of Neurology, Neurosurgery, and Psychiatry. 2018;**89**(9):949-954 available from: PM:29627773

[16] Hughes RA, Wijdicks EF, Benson E, Cornblath DR, Hahn AF, Meythaler JM, et al. Supportive care for patients with Guillain-Barre syndrome. Archives of Neurology. 2005;**62**(8):1194-1198 available from: PM:16087757

[17] Doets AY, Verboon C, van den Berg B, Harbo T, Cornblath DR, Willison HJ, et al. Regional variation of Guillain-Barre syndrome. Brain. 2018;**141**(10):2866-2877 available from: PM:30247567

[18] Chevret, S., Hughes, R.A., & Annane, D. 2017. Plasma exchange for Guillain-Barre syndrome. Cochrane. Database.Syst.Rev., 2, CD001798 available from: PM:28241090

[19] Hughes, R.A., Swan, A.V., & van Doorn, P.A. 2014. Intravenous immunoglobulin for Guillain-Barre syndrome. Cochrane.Database.Syst. Rev., 9, CD002063 available from: PM:25238327

[20] Davidson AI, Halstead SK, Goodfellow JA, Chavada G, Mallik A, Overell J, et al. Inhibition of complement in Guillain-Barre syndrome: The ICA-GBS study. J.Peripher.Nerv.Syst. 2017;**22**(1):4-12 available from: PM:27801990

[21] Misawa S, Kuwabara S, Sato Y, Yamaguchi N, Nagashima K, Katayama K, et al. Safety and efficacy of eculizumab in Guillain-Barre syndrome: A multicentre, double-blind, randomised phase 2 trial. Lancet Neurology. 2018;**17**(6):519-529 available from: PM:29685815

[22] Pritchard, J., Hughes, R.A., Hadden, R.D., & Brassington, R. 2016. Pharmacological treatment other than corticosteroids, intravenous immunoglobulin and plasma exchange for Guillain-Barre syndrome. Cochrane. Database.Syst.Rev., 11, CD008630 available from: PM:27846348

[23] Khan F, Amatya B. Rehabilitation interventions in patients with acute demyelinating inflammatory polyneuropathy: A systematic review. Eur.J.Phys.Rehabil.Med. 2012;**48**(3):507-522 available from: PM:22820829

[24] Khan F, Pallant JF, Amatya B, Ng L, Gorelik A, Brand C. Outcomes of high- and low-intensity rehabilitation programme for persons in chronic phase after Guillain-Barre syndrome: A randomized controlled trial. J.Rehabil. Med. 2011;**43**(7):638-646 available from: PM:21667009

[25] Demir SO, Koseoglu F. Factors associated with health-related quality of life in patients with severe Guillain-Barre syndrome. Disabil.Rehabil. 2008;**30**(8):593-599 available from: PM:17852306

[26] Gupta, A., Taly, A.B., Srivastava, A., & Murali, T. 2010. Guillain-Barre Syndrome–rehabilitation outcome, residual deficits and requirement of

lower limb orthosis for locomotion at 1 year follow-up. Disabil.Rehabil., 32, (23) 1897-1902 available from: PM:20331413

[27] Meythaler JM, DeVivo MJ, Braswell WC. Rehabilitation outcomes of patients who have developed Guillain-Barre syndrome. American Journal of Physical Medicine & Rehabilitation. 1997;**76**(5):411-419 available from: PM:9354496

[28] Nicholas R, Playford ED, Thompson AJ. A retrospective analysis of outcome in severe Guillain-Barre syndrome following combined neurological and rehabilitation management. Disabil.Rehabil. 2000;**22**(10):451-455 available from: PM:10950498

[29] Prada V, Massa F, Salerno A, Fregosi D, Beronio A, Serrati C, et al. Importance of intensive and prolonged rehabilitative treatment on the Guillain-Barre syndrome long-term outcome: A retrospective study. Neurol.Sci. 2019 available from: PM:31586288

[30] Medical Research Council. Aids to examination of the peripheral nervous system. London: HMSO. Memorandum No. 1976;**45**

[31] Hughes RA, Newsom-Davis JM, Perkin GD, Pierce JM. Controlled trial prednisolone in acute polyneuropathy. Lancet. 1978;**2**(8093):750-753 available from: PM:80682

[32] Simatos AN, Vincent PO, Yu BH, Bastien R, Sweeney A. Influence of exercise on patients with Guillain-Barre syndrome: A systematic review. Physiotherapy Canada. 2016;**68**(4):367-376 available from: PM:27904236

[33] Bussmann JB, Garssen MP, van Doorn PA, Stam HJ. Analysing the favourable effects of physical exercise: Relationships between physical fitness, fatigue and functioning in Guillain-Barre syndrome and chronic inflammatory demyelinating polyneuropathy. J.Rehabil.Med. 2007;**39**(2):121-125 available from: PM:17351693

[34] Garssen MP, Bussmann JB, Schmitz PI, Zandbergen A, Welter TG, Merkies IS, et al. Physical training and fatigue, fitness, and quality of life in Guillain-Barre syndrome and CIDP. Neurology. 2004;**63**(12):2393-2395 available from: PM:15623709

[35] Griffiths RD, Palmer TE, Helliwell T, MacLennan P, MacMillan RR. Effect of passive stretching on the wasting of muscle in the critically ill. Nutrition. 1995;**11**(5):428-432 available from: PM:8748193

[36] Reid CL, Campbell IT, Little RA. Muscle wasting and energy balance in critical illness. Clin.Nutr. 2004;**23**(2):273-280 available from: PM:15030968

[37] Maddocks, M., Gao, W., Higginson, I.J., & Wilcock, A. 2013. Neuromuscular electrical stimulation for muscle weakness in adults with advanced disease. Cochrane.Database.Syst. Rev. (1) CD009419 available from: PM:23440837

[38] Maffiuletti, N.A., Roig, M., Karatzanos, E., & Nanas, S. 2013. Neuromuscular electrical stimulation for preventing skeletal-muscle weakness and wasting in critically ill patients: A systematic review. BMC.Med., 11, 137 available from: PM:23701811

[39] Harbo T, Markvardsen LK, Hellfritzsch MB, Severinsen K, Nielsen JF, Andersen H. Neuromuscular electrical stimulation in early rehabilitation of Guillain-Barre syndrome: A pilot study. Muscle & Nerve. 2019;**59**(4):481-484 available from: PM:30549053

[40] El ML, Calmels P, Camdessanche JP, Gautheron V, Feasson L. Muscle

strength recovery in treated Guillain-Barre syndrome: A prospective study for the first 18 months after onset. American Journal of Physical Medicine & Rehabilitation. 2007;**86**(9):716-724 available from: PM:17709995

[41] Albiol-Perez S, Forcano-Garcia M, Munoz-TomasMT,Manzano-FernandezP, Solsona-Hernandez S, Mashat MA, et al. A novel virtual motor rehabilitation system for Guillain-Barre syndrome. Two single case studies. Methods Inf. Med. 2015;**54**(2):127-134 available from: PM:25609504

[42] Harbo T, Brincks J, Andersen H. Maximal isokinetic and isometric muscle strength of major muscle groups related to age, body mass, height, and sex in 178 healthy subjects. Eur.J.Appl. Physiol. 2012;**112**(1):267-275 available from: PM:21537927